50 Ways To Lose Your Blubber

Dr. Paul G. Varnas

Health Communications, Inc.
Deerfield Beach, Florida

Library of Congress Cataloging-in-Publication Data

Varnas, Paul G.
   Fifty ways to lose your blubber/by Paul G. Varnas.
     p. cm.
   Includes bibliographical references.
   ISBN 1-55874-229-8
   1. Reducing. I. Title. II. Title: 50 Ways to lose your blubber.
RM222.2.V37 1992
613.2′5—dc20   92-4903
                                                    CIP

©1993 Paul G. Varnas
ISBN 1-55874-229-8

Publisher: Health Communications, Inc.
               3201 S.W. 15th Street
               Deerfield Beach, Florida 33442-8190

Cover design by Barbara Bergman

To Our Readers:

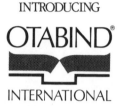

This book is dedicated to
my wife, Sharon, who has literally
stuck with me through
thick and thin.

A special thanks
to Lisa Moro, who
encouraged, edited and
worked for this book.

Contents

The 50 Ways vii

Preface ix

Introduction xi

Section A: Motivation 1

Section B: Activity 25

Section C: Controlling What You Eat 49

Section D: Limiting Caloric Intake The Right Way 93

Section E: Health Considerations 115

Section F: Miscellaneous 135

Bibliography 151

The 50 Ways

1. Read This Book xvii
2. Lose The Guilt 2
3. Set Goals 3
4. Visualize 5
5. Enjoy The Process 7
6. Keep A Food Diary 9
7. Lose Weight With A Friend 11
8. Avoid "All-Or-Nothing" Thinking 12
9. Don't Be In A Hurry 14
10. Reward Yourself 15
11. Take This One Day At A Time 16
12. You Don't "Have To" Do Anything 17
13. Don't Get Hung Up On Your Day-To-Day Weight 19
14. Keep Trying, Even Though You Feel As If You've Failed .. 21
15. Keep Trying, Even Though You Feel As If
    You've Succeeded 23
16. Exercise, Exercise, Exercise 27
17. Make Yourself Work Harder 41
18. Destroy Your Television 43
19. Get Busy, Stop Being Sedentary 46
20. Don't Diet Or Get Hung Up On Calories 50

21. Absolutely Avoid Refined Sugar 56
22. Don't Starve Yourself 59
23. Eat If You're Hungry 61
24. Eat Whole Grains 63
25. Don't Get Hung Up On Nutritional Fads And
    Buzz Words 67
26. Learn How To Read Labels And Choose Your Food 71
27. Eat Lots Of Fresh Fruit And Vegetables 85
28. Absolutely Avoid Commercially Fried Foods 87
29. Buy Organically Grown Foods Whenever Possible 88
30. Learn To Control Cravings 90
31. Eat Slowly. Chew Your Food Thoroughly 96
32. Learn To Like Plain Foods 98
33. Don't Clean Your Plate 100
34. Don't Clean Someone Else's Plate 102
35. Don't Eat If You're Not Hungry 103
36. Beware Of Triggers 104
37. Eat Only At The Table 106
38. Wait A Few Minutes Before Taking Seconds 107
39. Eat Vegetarian One Day Each Week 108
40. Leave The Table As Soon As You Are Finished 109
41. Don't Sample Foods While Cooking 110
42. Don't Do Anything Else While Eating 111
43. Control Yourself In Situations Where You Are Likely
    To Overeat 112
44. Be Aware If You Have Digestive Problems 116
45. Be Aware Of The Possibility Of Food Allergies 122
46. Get Help If You Need It 127
47. Expect To Feel Good 129
48. Drink Water 131
49. Avoid Common Mistakes 136
50. Design Your Own Program 143

Preface

With bookshelves filled with diet and fitness books — diets based on the immune system, stimulating the metabolism, eliminating fat and all kinds of "miracle" diets — why another book about losing weight? The reason is that, in spite of all of the money and effort that goes into weight loss, surprisingly few people actually lose weight and keep it off. It seems as if there are only a few dozen people who have ever lost and kept off a significant amount of weight. I suspect that they're all being held prisoner by Jenny Craig, only to be let out to do the occasional commercial.

Most diet books give you a pamphlet's worth of information expanded to 200 or 300 pages with authoritarian diatribe. Conventional wisdom dictates that the American public would rather have a simple idea spoon-fed to them. Unfortunately health and physiology are not simple subjects.

This is not a diet book. There are no gimmicks for weight loss. This book will, however, show you how to change your habits permanently to become healthy.

Although losing weight may be your primary concern, you must realize that becoming your ideal weight is only one aspect of being healthy. Just being thin isn't good enough. If it were, we'd all be anxiously awaiting Madonna's new health and exercise video. Just think of becoming your ideal weight as a nice side effect of getting healthy.

This book will help you understand why changes need to be made, why some unhealthy habits are so compelling and how to adopt new healthy habits without feeling a strong sense of sacrifice.

By reading this you will learn about your own physiology. It will teach you why you crave certain foods and how to control those cravings. I've tried to anticipate the problems you will have in trying to become thinner and healthier and offer you ways to overcome those problems. You will not only lose the weight, but you will learn to keep it off. You should be able to lose weight without feeling hungry, tired or irritable.

Introduction

IT CAN HAPPEN TO ANYONE

Everyone who is overweight has a story about how he or she became heavy. Some have been heavy all of their lives. Some have started by trying to lose five or ten pounds and over the years have yo-yoed themselves up to a size 18. Some have had babies and were unable to lose the weight afterward. That's how my problem began.

Two years ago I was the picture of health and fitness. I weighed 170 pounds — my weight in high school. I worked out every day, had good endurance and strength and was even becoming more flexible.

One morning I woke up to find myself 45 pounds overweight. I'd had surgery a few months earlier, which interrupted my work-out schedule. Three weeks after the surgery the doctor gave me a clean bill of health and said to start exercising again. Like most patients, I ignored him.

But it was my wife who helped me turn from Adonis to John Madden. She had been systematically shrinking my clothes for months. That was just the beginning. She did something that guaranteed I'd become overweight: She became pregnant. (I guess I did get *some* exercise after the surgery.)

Anyone married to a pregnant woman soon realizes he is at the mercy of her blood sugar swings. He quickly learns that this irrational being he lives with, the one prone to outbursts of anger and sorrow, can be magically placed into a euphoric state by a pint of Haagen Dazs ice cream. This is the greatest discovery an expectant father can make. Haagen Dazs: Marital bliss in a carton. No wonder they don't advertise.

I built a small altar in our doorway. When I came home, I'd leave the ice cream on it and wait. When it was gone, I knew it was safe to enter the house.

Unfortunately, it didn't take long for me to realize that Haagen Dazs put me into a euphoric state as well. It was like *The Days of Wine And Roses* done in ice cream. We'd lie next to each other in a near diabetic coma with an empty carton of macadamia nut brittle between us. For every bowl she had, I had two. For every pound she gained, I gained a pound and a half.

We live in Chicago where you can have any kind of food delivered at almost any time. Some places will even stop and pick up a six pack and a video for you. Even the grocery stores deliver. All this and cable television. We were in heaven.

The woman teaching our childbirth class said the fact that I was getting so heavy meant I was a sensitive husband. We were so thrilled that we celebrated with pizza. But I guess the instructor really meant that I kept my pregnant wife from feeling fat and heavy by becoming fatter and heavier.

Then came the birth of our daughter, the happiest day of our lives. My wife lost half of the weight she had gained in one evening. I had donuts at the nurses' station. At least the donuts didn't cause me to gain any more weight that evening. Standing at the foot of a bed yelling "push" for 12 hours burns up a fair number of calories.

The baby never slept, nor did we. We didn't get out much but I did take care of my new family. Realizing that a nursing mother needs a lot of calcium and protein, I ordered pizza almost every night, usually with root beer, just to keep her blood sugar up (better safe than sorry with that blood sugar). I forgot where the gym was.

My wife has one of those magic metabolisms; she can eat anything and not gain weight. She still has clothes from junior high school (they're even back in style now). Two months after the baby was born she was back to wearing her original size three. I, on the other hand, ballooned up to 215 pounds: 45 pounds higher than my ideal weight and 30 pounds more than the weight that used to panic me into doing something about it. I had to lose 30 pounds to become what I used to consider fat.

My life had become a blur of ice cream, Doritos, dirty diapers and "America's Funniest Home Videos." We even set up a camera and waited for the couch to collapse, hoping to pick up an extra ten grand. To our surprise it didn't, although it sagged about a foot lower where I usually sat.

I felt lousy; I was tired all of the time. Not much besides eating was pleasurable. I didn't like going out because none of my clothes fit. I wore surgical scrubs around the house and big baggy Hawaiian shirts when we went out — anything large and loose that kept me from confronting my weight.

The irony of all this is that I'm a chiropractor and a large portion of my practice consists of giving nutritional advice. I knew what I needed to do, but I just couldn't get motivated enough to do it. I was too tired, too busy, too whatever excuse I could think of to keep from doing anything about it. I shifted the emphasis of my practice to bad backs. At least I was credible in that area. So don't feel bad. Anyone can get fat. There is something very compelling about eating junk food and being sedentary. Eating empty calories tends to make you want to eat more empty calories. Foods with empty calories are foods that have sugar, starch, fat and little else. These foods are deficient in vitamins and minerals and eating them is just a habit that's easier to break than you think. The hard part is getting started, but you've done that already by getting this book and reading this far.

There are really only two ways to get fat: eating too much of the wrong things and not eating enough of the right things. There are junk food junkies who are fat and there are people who don't eat very much and can't seem to lose their extra weight. It doesn't matter which category you fall into, this book can help you.

Other than the time someone painted me silver and wrote "Goodyear" on my side, becoming this fat has been a positive experience. There is a big difference between having to lose five or ten pounds and needing to lose nearly 50. I now understand what my heavy patients go through.

When you're 45 pounds overweight, you don't feel very good. It's hard to get motivated. This is why bookstores sell so many programs that stress a single angle such as, "All you have to do is stay away from carbohydrates" or "All you have to do is stay away from fat" or "All you have to do is eat grapefruit after every meal." You want something simple that allows you to lose the weight and get it over with. Unfortunately that never works.

DIETERS TEND TO BLAME THEMSELVES

Dieters tend to blame themselves for their failures. But the reason most diets fail is not the fault of the dieter. There is a plethora of oversimplification and misinformation, if not outright deceit, in the area of weight loss.

A quick fix is easy to sell to people who are obese or who are yo-yo dieters. It seems as if the more failures dieters experience, the more extreme the programs they are willing to try. Perhaps frustration drives them to desperate measures. Perhaps it is the hope of finding that magic program that will take the weight off quickly. Making moderate changes takes time. If you have 40 or 50 pounds to lose, you're looking at six months (or more) on a very strict diet. Six months of being hungry, six months of giving up the foods you love and six months of knowing that six months probably isn't enough. No wonder there are so many extreme programs that find takers.

I have a relative who went on a medically supervised fasting program. It cost her a couple of thousand dollars. She drank a protein and vitamin concoction and had regular medical checkups to make sure she wasn't having any side effects, such as kidney failure or death. She was not exercising and received nothing in the way of dietary fiber. She lost 62 pounds in about four months. She said she felt great and it was better than dieting because food was not an issue. However, when she stopped using the program, she went right back to her old eating habits. As a result, she gained most of her weight back and will probably gain the rest of it in time. Oprah Winfrey made a program like this famous before she started regaining her weight.

Most people view weight loss as a temporary, unpleasant task which they will abandon as soon as they reach their target weight. *What is really needed is a permanent change of habits.* By that, I mean a gradual change to healthy ways of eating and increased activity, not a diet that lasts forever.

Fast weight loss is interpreted by the body as starvation. It will slow down its metabolism to conserve calories. Very often after a strict diet, a dieter will become ravenously hungry — even minor self-control seems impossible. This is why many people are successful on a diet, but fail to stay with the maintenance program.

Weight loss is a crisis that your body works very hard to avoid. Our physiologies are not prepared to deal with modern civilization and its empty calories, refined carbohydrates, hydrogenated fats and wide variety of food additives.

Evolution is a slow process. You still own the body of a prehistoric hunter-gatherer who didn't know where his or her next meal was coming from. A little fat was good for survival. Prehistoric humans did not have Cheetos and Twix Bars. They ate whole foods, things that grew from the ground and, occasionally, a wild animal. They had no labor-saving devices, they walked everywhere. Chances are they didn't get very fat. A little extra fat meant they had some energy reserve when it was needed. Since obesity wasn't a problem, their bodies valued fat and tried to hang on to it. Your physiology isn't much different from that of prehistoric humans. Obesity is a new problem, a disease of civilization, so our bodies don't have built-in mechanisms to deal with it. When we try to lose weight, we are often thwarted by our own survival instincts.

Sounds pretty grim: Diets don't work and your body actually likes to be fat. Actually it's not that bad, just something you've probably suspected all along: *Dieting is an unnatural act.* You can still lose weight but you just won't do it by dieting.

Stop blaming yourself for past failures. The last time you stuck with a diet for a week or so only to break down and take the staff of a Dunkin' Donuts hostage until you could finish off their inventory wasn't your fault. It wasn't your lack of willpower — it was a diet that wasn't appropriate to your needs.

You can learn to lose weight by first understanding how your body works. In 1918, Dr. Lulu Hunt Peters wrote the book *Diet*

And Health. In it she presented the concept of counting calories. A calorie is a measurement of energy (much like the BTU used to rate furnaces). In nutrition, it is the amount of heat required to raise the temperature of one liter of water one degree centigrade. A pound of fat contains 3,500 calories. Dr. Peters suggested a diet of 1,200 calories per day for weight loss and 15 calories per pound per day for weight maintenance. For instance, a 200-pound person maintains his or her weight with 3,000 calories per day. It is an idea that has endured for years because there is a lot of value in knowing the caloric content of foods.

But the simple idea of eating fewer calories than you burn up is further complicated by other physiologic considerations such as basal metabolism, digestion, how many calories are actually absorbed and food allergies. Why else would statistics show that Americans are consuming fewer calories per capita than they did earlier in this century, yet their average weight continues to rise? *If you are going to lose weight, you will have to learn how your body works, use a little discipline and get motivated.*

This book will help you design your own successful program to lose weight. There is information on:

- Physiology — the way your body works
- Possible health problems contributing to your inability to lose weight
- Tricks to help you change habits
- Ways to motivate yourself

Designing your own program will take a little more effort than having a canned program that tells you what and when to eat. You will, however, be more successful if you learn a little basic physiology and make your own choices than if you blindly follow a program designed for a mythical average person.

1

Read This Book

You will be designing your own weight loss program, so be sure to read everything before you decide which changes you are going to make first.

There are no gimmicks in this book. No panacea or new revolutionary method for you to lose weight. Just common sense and information that will help you understand why you have trouble losing weight.

Read this book, and reread it at some point during your program. You will begin to understand how your body works and how to apply that knowledge to losing weight. If you've had problems disciplining yourself in the past, you will learn ways to make it easy on yourself.

Presented here are 50 ways to lose weight. They fall into six categories:

- Motivation
- Activity
- Controlling what you eat
- Limiting caloric intake the right way
- Health considerations
- Miscellaneous.

Motivation

Motivation is the most important thing in losing weight. It's hard to get motivated to change your habits. Smokers have trouble quitting. Many of us have trouble giving up certain foods. And some people can't discipline themselves to get more organized. Change is hard unless your reasons for change are stronger than those for staying the same. You can increase your desire to change, thus improving your chances of success, by doing what is listed in this section. In order to change, you have to become motivated.

Becoming thin and feeling good have to be real to you. If you've been heavy for a long time or have failed at many diets, you may have a built-in sense of failure. You need to *want* to change and *expect* to be successful. You also need to take steps to ensure that you will stay on your program. The items listed in this section will help you get excited about losing weight and keep you interested in developing a workable program.

Lose The Guilt

People who have dieted and failed tend to feel guilty or at least blame themselves for not having enough willpower. Don't blame yourself and don't anticipate failure this time. If you expect to fail, you become a victim of self-fulfilling prophecy. You'll be more likely to eat that box of cookies late at night if you have an attitude such as, "Why bother trying, I never lose weight anyway." Your mind is a very powerful tool. Expect failure and that's what you'll get.

Chances are that you've dieted before and lost weight only to gain it back. You probably know more people who have dieted unsuccessfully than people who have lost weight and kept it off.

People who can't lose weight tend to think they lack willpower, but the truth is they have more willpower than they think. I have a patient who told me that over the years, he's lost almost 200 pounds through dieting. That really took willpower and is not diminished by the fact that he's gained about 220 pounds during the same time.

You're not heavy because you lack a strong will. When you begin to understand how your physiology works, you'll know that the failure to lose weight is not your fault but the fault of the methods you were using. So don't feel guilty if you have been unable to lose weight in the past.

Set Goals

In order to lose weight, you have to *decide* to lose it. That doesn't mean that you'll *try* to lose it. Make a conscious decision and *believe* that you will be successful. Set a weight goal and write it down. If you have no idea what your ideal weight should be, you can have a body composition analysis done that will tell you your percentages of fat and lean tissue. Many health clubs and physicians' offices have devices to do this. Males should have about 16 percent body fat and females should have about 23 percent. Usually there is a setting on the machine that will tell you your ideal weight, although most of us already have an idea of what we should weigh.

When you write your goal down, don't just stop with the weight. How big around should your waist, hips and thighs be? What size should you be wearing? Get a very clear idea of what you want your size and weight to be.

You can set a timetable if you like. It's not absolutely necessary. Some people will feel pressured by a time frame, others will be motivated by it. If you do set time goals, be realistic. Don't plan to lose five pounds per week. You'll only set yourself up for disappointment. Remember: *Rapid weight loss is the exception rather than the rule.*

If you're in a hurry, intense exercise will serve you better than strict caloric restriction. Prisoners in the concentration camps during World War II were fed only 800 calories per day, which is a starvation diet even by Dr. Peter's standards. The prisoners lost an average of only two pounds per week.

If you're really dedicated to losing weight, and you don't encounter any special problems, you can learn to lose approximately a pound per week. There are ways to lose the weight a little faster, but it is more likely to stay off if you take your time.

If you are losing less than a pound per week, don't worry. Consistency is what is important. If you want to lose weight a little faster, try making some of the changes you haven't yet made or try increasing your physical activity.

If the changes recommended here seem overwhelming at first and it is difficult for you to imagine doing everything listed, your goal may include a timetable to implement the various changes. Everyone is different. Some may want to completely overhaul their life-styles as soon as possible. Some will view their bad habits as old friends they are reluctant to give up. No matter what type of person you are, you will lose weight. Believe that. As long as you are trying to change your habits consistently, you can't miss.

☐☐☐ *Read your goals every day; get excited about them. Get excited about being at the weight you want to be. Every day reaffirm your commitment to losing weight and becoming the person you want to be.*

Visualize

Think of this as time spent programming yourself to be thin. Take about 15 minutes each day and visualize yourself as the person you want to become. This is very important. This is where your self-control will come from. Don't just think about your weight as a number. Make the image real. What size are you wearing? What does your stomach look like? How do you look in a bathing suit? (Please don't send pictures, these are just rhetorical questions.)

Fill in as many details as possible. Imagine the kinds of things people say to you. Picture your social life. How does your spouse (boyfriend, girlfriend) feel about the new you? How is your energy level? What kinds of things do you spend your time doing? Get emotional while doing this. Really feel how it is to be your best self. Get excited about how good you feel and how good you look.

Many people claim they don't visualize well. Everyone visualizes. Try not to see a purple gorilla. You see, your mind already formed a picture, in spite of yourself. It's hard not to visualize. Just because you don't close your eyes and see vivid technicolor pictures doesn't mean you can't visualize.

If seeing with your mind's eye doesn't come easily to you, just practice. You'll get better at it. You can also use other senses. Hear what people are saying. Feel what your emotional state is. Feel what it is like to put your hands in your lap. Feel what it is like to have a lap. Feel what it is like to put your hands on your hips (and have the fingers actually point down for a change). Smell the perfume (or after shave) of that sexy new person in your life. Feel the fear for your life when your spouse learns of this. The more senses you involve, the more vivid the image will be and the more motivated you will become.

The energy you put into visualizing will help you overcome bad habits. You can picture your ideal self having a total disdain for chocolate, ice cream, potato chips, midnight snacking or whatever habits you have that now keep you fat. The importance of this cannot be overstressed. Regular visualizing will put you in control of your habits.

━━━━━ *The more you think about how wonderful it will feel to become thin and healthy, the more you will want to do to achieve your weight goals. Spending enough time and energy on it and becoming that ideal person will become more important to you than that pizza during the football game, ice cream before bed or finishing off the 14 pounds of cookies you baked for your child's school.*

5

Enjoy The Process

A diet is a short-term, unpleasant task which is abandoned when a weight goal is reached. No one ever enjoys dieting and few people are a success at it. You will be more successful if the process of losing weight is pleasant.

You need to change your eating habits and life-style permanently. In order to be successful, you must like the changes you make. Re-educating yourself about eating and activity will work where diets fail.

Diets are never tailored to the individual. Everyone is different and there are many variables, but few diets take those into consideration. How big you are, how lousy you feel, whether or not you're in reasonably good aerobic condition, what kind of medical problems you now have, how slow your metabolism is or how active you are will all play a role in how things will go. No expert knows what is best for you and not every friend who's read Adele Davis is an expert. You can get advice on losing weight from magazines, books, people in health-food stores and your dear Aunt Edna who "reads a lot." What helped Aunt Edna's neighbor's daughter, Dolores, lose weight may not exactly work for you. Maybe the program is too restrictive. Perhaps it just is not appropriate for you.

If you are overweight (a safe assumption if you're reading this), there is a reason for it. How you eat, what you eat, how active you are or the general state of your health has something to do with it. It stands to reason that if you change what is wrong and don't change back, you will lose the weight and keep it off. If the changes you make are unpleasant, you eventually will go back to your old habits and ultimately will fail. So take it at your own pace.

You say, "But I love to eat donuts and Pepsi for breakfast. I'll never enjoy giving that up." That may be true now. Forcing yourself to give it up will never work. You must teach yourself how not to like it or how to enjoy an alternative — a healthy breakfast, for instance. This is where visualizing comes into play. This book will also teach you some tricks to bring your cravings under control. If you truly are tired of being so big that you have your own personal zip code, you will be able to change habits like this that keep you fat. Because habits are learned, if you can learn to like something, you can also learn not to like something else. It is easier than you think to reprogram yourself.

As you read some of these suggestions, you may say to yourself, "I'll never give that up" or "I can't do that." Don't worry about that right now. Begin by making the changes that come easily to you. The more changes you make, the easier the others will become. If you make it too unpleasant for yourself, you won't change permanently. Consistency is more important than speed.

Don't worry, you won't have to be psyching yourself up continually to keep on your program. The improvements you make will be their own reward. You will feel so much better than before that you won't want to go back to your old habits. Eating properly is a matter of developing new habits and tastes. You will have a lot more energy than ever before. You will not be hungry.

This book will teach you why you have cravings and how to get rid of them. You will be able to apply the information not only to reach the weight you desire, but also to have the health and energy you deserve. The weight loss may take a long time, but you will notice these other benefits much sooner.

Set your own pace, be comfortable with the changes you make. This is fun. You're going to be thin and feel great. Get excited about that.

Keep A Food Diary

Even before you start your program, write down everything you eat during a two-week period. Your results may surprise you. Many people don't realize how much junk they eat until they write down all the food they consume.

If you're really ambitious, you can figure out how much fat, calories, protein and carbohydrates you're consuming. There's a book by Helen Church and Jean Pennington called *Food Values*. It lists calories, fat, carbohydrates, protein, cholesterol and even the vitamin and mineral content of different foods.

The Center for Science in the Public Interest is a nonprofit organization. The center produces a monthly newsletter that is worth getting. It will teach you a lot about the contents of foods and how labels can be misleading. It also provides good general information about nutrition. Write to them at:

1875 Connecticut Ave. N.W.

Washington, DC 20009-5728

The book or the computer program can help you to get a clear idea of how many calories you now consume. You will find out if you're getting too much fat, too much protein, too many carbohydrates or not enough vitamins. Getting a clear picture of what is wrong with the way you're eating will make it easy to change your habits.

Once you begin your program, writing down the food you eat will help you keep on it. You won't want to write down eating that two-pound bag of fried pork rinds or the box of cherry bonbons in your diary. The food diary will also show you if you're getting enough fresh vegetables, water and other essential foods.

Keeping a dietary diary will help motivate you. You will be able to keep track of how much you've improved as your program progresses. A dietary diary will help reinforce your determination to stay with your program. You can also write down your weight goal and keep track of your weight in it.

Lose Weight With A Friend

Losing weight is much easier if you're doing it with one or more of your friends than by yourself. You can offer each other support and encouragement by talking each other out of stashing Little Debbie cakes in the bottom of the closet. You may even find a little friendly competition helpful. You can bet on who will lose the next five pounds fastest. You can also share low-calorie recipes and other good food ideas.

You can even exercise together. This really is helpful because you will end up taking turns with your friend. One of you will be an enthusiastic pain in the neck while the other will want to sit this one out. It's a great way to ensure that you'll exercise, even when you don't feel like it.

▭ *The support offered by another person trying to accomplish the same goal will help motivate you. This is what makes Weight Watchers and Overeaters Anonymous so attractive to many dieters.*

Avoid "All-Or-Nothing" Thinking

There is a ritual to dieting. At the start, most dieters follow every direction with the zealousness of a Shiite. That's good. I hope you follow my advice that thoroughly because it will make you feel great. There is a problem, however, with being too zealous. If you break down temporarily and have a donut, a bag of potato chips or a two-pound box of Godiva chocolates, you tend to think that you've failed.

This is a habit picked up from dieting. You feel that either you're on the diet or you're not. Even worse, many dieters feel they might as well eat sweets, fried foods or any other kind of junk food that appeals to them since they've "blown the diet anyway." This is not a good idea.

If you've failed at many diets, your first indiscretion may make you think that you've blown it or that you'll never lose weight, but don't worry. Your dietary diary will help you here. If you compare your eating habits to the two weeks prior to the time you started your program, even with the chocolates you had in a moment of weakness, you'll probably find that your new habits are much better than they used to be. Just consistently try to improve and don't worry about the momentary ups and downs.

In school, 90 percent is still an "A," so even if you lapse into a few old habits 10 percent of the time, you'll still lose weight. (Since 78 percent is a C-, try to do a little better than that, otherwise we'll have to line up my old grade-school principal to give you a little grief on Friday afternoons.)

Going back to your old dietary habits may make you feel lousy and that may add to your discouragement. If you've stopped eating sugar, for example, going back to it will bring back the blood sugar swings and the cravings. Just make sure you understand that. Going back to your program may be a little difficult after a lapse in discipline, and it may take a day or two before you feel as good as you do when you are really watching what you eat. During that time, it is very easy to beat yourself up about how weak-willed you are. Realize that it's just the sugar talking. Noticing how you feel when you cheat may help motivate you. Most of us would rather feel good than indulge in dietary indiscretions once we realize that it's our eating habits that make us feel bad.

A little lapse is not going to ruin all the effort you've put into your program. Rather than becoming discouraged, work out a little harder than before or eat vegetarian the next day. The main thing is not to feel guilty, give up and go back to your old habits.

There are going to be holidays, birthdays, outings, dates and other events that you won't be able to (or should want to) avoid. It's not that big a deal to have birthday cake. Enjoy yourself. Then go back to your program the next day.

Don't Be In A Hurry

It took time for you to put on the weight. It will take time for you to take it off. There are no quick fixes. Actually there are plenty of them, but they don't work. The key to this program is for you to change your habits permanently. This will take time. You have to be comfortable with the changes or you will go back to your old habits.

It may be tempting to combine parts of an old diet or substitute meals with protein drinks while you are doing this. You may lose a few pounds and that will inspire you to try to speed up the process. Don't get into a hurry. All of the information you need to lose weight is contained right here. As I write this, I'm 20 pounds lighter than I was when I started. I even lost three pounds over the holidays staying with my in-laws. In case you're wondering, yes, I cheated. But there are ways to minimize the damage. We'll cover that later.

It isn't absolutely necessary that you do everything listed in this book right away. The more you do, though, the faster you will achieve your goal. Start with what comes easy to you, then add other things later. Proceed at your own pace.

Reward Yourself

If you have a little something to look forward to every time you lose another five or ten pounds, it will motivate you. Get a massage, go to the theater, take a trip, take a mental-health day off from work, go to Europe, buy jewelry, go out on the town or have your nose fixed.

Do something that makes you feel as if you are indulging yourself, although I don't recommend a hot fudge sundae or a pitcher of beer.

Take This One Day At A Time

This attitude works for alcoholics so it'll work for you. One day you find yourself fantasizing about having a hot fudge sundae, smothered in whipped cream and nuts, until it crowds out all your other thoughts. You begin to salivate and think of nothing else. At this point, don't say to yourself, "I can never have another sundae again," as you try to find something with which to slash your wrists. Just put off having it or decide not to have it today. Don't think in terms of "never." It's too overwhelming and will intensify the temptation and sense of sacrifice.

⬜▬ *Every day is a new one, just renew your decision for the day. You won't suffer from chocolate withdrawal or a Pepsi deficiency. It's just a habit. It's easier to break than you think, and it will get easier as time goes by. Also realize that today is when you are losing weight, not tomorrow or next week.*

You Don't "Have To" Do Anything

This is *your* program. You are doing this to look and feel better. What you eat or don't eat is entirely up to you. Never say to yourself, "I can't have that case of Twinkies because I'm on a diet."

You are not on a diet; you're changing some habits to become thin and healthy. What you eat is your choice. A case of Twinkies will make it take longer for you to reach your goal, but the world won't end because of it. If you get strong cravings, maybe you aren't eating frequently enough, or have food allergies or digestive problems.

Just because you've read this book, agreed with what it says and have decided that you want to change your eating habits, doesn't mean that certain foods won't appeal to you emotionally. You see chocolate or perhaps some fried snack food and remember how much you enjoyed eating it. Saying to yourself that you can't eat it isn't good enough. Refusing to eat it takes willpower. Willpower is wanting something and denying yourself. It isn't a very effective tool for controlling your behavior. You won't be very successful with this if you feel that you are denying yourself. This is why visualizing is so important. It will help you to stop reacting emotionally to certain foods.

You're going for long-term change here. It is important that you not feel deprived. Take the time to solve these problems and bring your cravings under control. There are lots of ways to do this and they're covered in the chapter "Controlling What You Eat." Before you finish this book, you will know why you have cravings and how to bring them under control.

☐══════ *The issue is not whether you can or cannot have the candy, pop, pizza, carton of donuts or side of beef, but whether eating it is more important to you than reaching your goal. The choice is yours.*

Don't Get Hung Up On Your Day-To-Day Weight

Don't weigh yourself every day; do it once a week. Your weight often varies a pound or two during the course of a day. If you are allergic to a certain food and eat it, you may even gain a couple of pounds. If you have a temporary gain one day, you may become discouraged.

If you are doing a lot of exercising, especially if you are lifting weights, you may actually gain weight. You will develop more muscle from working out and muscle weighs more than fat. Even aerobic workouts will cause you to gain more muscle mass so it is possible to lose fat and gain muscle by following your program, causing you to have a net gain in weight.

If you've plateaued, stay with the program. Don't be discouraged. There may be areas where you need improvement. It's a good time to forgo those enriched rolls you've been avoiding giving up. You may need more vegetables or exercise. You may be regularly eating a food that you're allergic to. You may have digestive problems. Your metabolism may be slow from being on several different diets. Increase your activity and see where else you can improve.

Use Other Measurements

When you begin your program, you may want to measure your waist, hips and thighs. Very often you will lose inches but not pounds. Having these other measurements to mark your progress will help keep you motivated when there isn't much weight loss. I frequently have patients tell me they haven't lost much weight but their clothes are looser. If you can find a way to have your body composition analyzed, you will get a better idea of how you are doing.

There are several ways to get a body composition analysis. The most accurate is through hydrostatic weighing, which involves being dipped into a tank to see how much water you displace. (They used Lake Michigan for me.) Hydrostatic weighing is usually used as a research tool and isn't generally available. There are skin-fold measurements, but these are not very accurate and results will vary from tester to tester. There are electronic devices which measure the body's resistance to an electric charge. These aren't bad, but there is a certain amount of error involved with them.

In my office I have one of the electronic devices. It is used to find a person's target weight and to keep track of how much fat he or she is losing versus lean body mass. Many health clubs and physicians' offices will do these measurements for you.

Keep Trying, Even Though
You Feel As If You've Failed

You've had a *Lost Weekend* and wake up in the gutter next to Ray Milland, your face smeared with chocolate, your breath reeking of Doritos. The last thing you remember saying was, "Oh well, it's my birthday, I'll just have one dessert." You realize that was eight days ago. The sugar cane futures market has been skyrocketing since you've gone on your little binge. Your memory is a hazy blur of Hostess Ding Dongs and peanut M&Ms. You feel bloated and ashamed. You want to quit. Don't. A lot of the weight and girth you've gained is water weight. A few days of correct eating and exercise and you'll see that the damage was not disastrous.

You can actually go off your program through no fault of your own. You may catch a cold, get the flu or injure yourself and be unable to exercise for a while. When you begin to feel better, you may be discouraged and feel as if you are starting all over again. Other things, such as vacations, family emergencies and holidays, may also interrupt your program. If circumstances keep you from following an exercise program or for some reason you are not eating as well as you should, at least continue to visualize and keep your weight goal clear in your mind. Doing this will make it easier for you to resume your program when your circumstances change.

You may even lose interest in trying to lose weight for a while, especially if you've lost 10 or 15 pounds and you still have a way to go. Give yourself permission to stop trying to *lose* weight. Concentrate instead on keeping off the weight you've lost. You can allow yourself to plateau for weeks or even months. Just maintain your weight and keep in mind that you will ultimately reach your goal. You can resume your program in earnest when you are ready.

▭ *Even if you've stayed away from your program for quite a while, keep trying. With each successive effort your new better habits will become more ingrained.*

Keep Trying, Even Though You Feel As If You've Succeeded

Although it will be tempting to drop the program and celebrate with a case of root beer and a truck load of pork rinds once you reach your target weight, don't abandon the program. Continue to weigh yourself every week. I know someone who has lost over 60 pounds on a medically supervised fast and has been slam dunking hot fudge sundaes ever since he went off the program. He's not entirely to blame. That program was so extreme that it had his body thinking it was starving.

It's part of the dieter's mentality to quit when the weight is off. Diets are unpleasant and you look forward to stopping and being able to "eat normally" again. Unfortunately, for many, eating normally means donuts for breakfast, hot dogs for lunch and ice cream before bed. This is one reason why so many diets fail.

Following the advice in this book will have you taking the changes slowly so you won't have that problem. You will develop a new way of life on your way to becoming thin. When you reach your ideal weight you should still be concerned about your health. The habits you pick up losing the weight will help you to live longer and feel better.

You do have to be careful that you don't slip slowly back to your old eating habits. Attaining your goal may make you complacent. Just keep exercising and weighing yourself. If your weight creeps up five pounds, become more disciplined with your habits.

B

Activity

Being active will be much more helpful to you in your quest to lose weight than eating less will. If you are sedentary, it will be next to impossible to lose weight and keep it off. Daily exercise is important, but you must also try to be more active in your day-to-day life.

In this section, I've provided a lot of information about how many calories are burned by various activities. The benefits of exercise and of being more active actually go beyond the figures that I've provided. An active person who exercises regularly will burn more calories at rest than a sedentary person. That is, he or she will have a higher basal metabolic rate.

There are many overweight people who don't eat much. They may actually consume fewer calories than thin people. ("I can't understand how you can eat so much and stay so thin. I just look at food and I gain weight.")

Frequent dieting will often slow down your basal metabolic rate, making the dieter fatigued, miserable and unable to lose weight. The best way to remedy this problem is by being active. Increased activity helps your body to produce enzymes that will actually aid in breaking down fat. You will also undergo hormonal changes that will increase your basal metabolic rate causing you not only to lose weight easier, but to have more energy as well.

Exercise, Exercise, Exercise

With the possible exception of visualizing, this is the most important thing you can do to lose weight. If you both exercise and visualize you will begin to notice results, even if you don't do much to change how you eat. You can exercise without dieting and lose weight more effectively and more permanently than you can by dieting without exercise. Often when you diet without exercising, most weight loss results from muscle breaking down. Actually, dieting without exercising may ultimately cause you to gain weight. It is important to exercise in a way that maximizes the burning of body fat.

Dieting alone is not enough. Exercise will increase your production of thyroxine that increases the rate at which you burn calories. Thus your metabolism will speed up. Exercise also will help you to produce enzymes that will enable you to mobilize fat and break it down.

You need to burn 3,500 calories more than you consume to lose one pound of fat. Thirty minutes of swimming (slow crawl for someone weighing 170 pounds) per day burns about 300 calories. If you change nothing else in your diet or in how active you are, that's one pound of fat lost in 12 days, or 30 pounds of fat lost in one year. There is an added bonus: Exercise increases your resting metabolism, so you will burn more calories even when you're not exercising.

Heavy people burn more calories than thin people making the same amount of effort. So take heart, if you're so fat that NASA has to know where you are before they make calculations for a launch, you'll really burn a lot of calories by exercising.

If you're extremely overweight, the thought of exercise is abhorrent. This was something I didn't understand before I became big enough to have several small chiropractors orbiting me. I would tell my heavy patients to exercise without understanding how hard it would be for them to start working out.

When I became 45 pounds overweight, I understood what it meant to be in love with my couch: to enjoy watching *Dobie Gillis* reruns and have all my food delivered. Our exercycle sat in the corner of the room, all alone with cobwebs on it. I'd look at it and just the thought of using it would be painful. All of that heavy breathing and muscle soreness — I was tired, my joints were stiff and the seat was too hard. It was nothing like the nice soft couch already contour-shaped to my rear end. Besides, I didn't have to clean cobwebs off of the couch to use it. The handles on my exercycle move so you can work the upper body. It's a good idea, but it left nowhere to put the Doritos. Exercise was unthinkable. But I had to begin. It was either that or invest in wider door frames.

During the time you spend visualizing, you can psyche yourself up to start to exercise.

The key to getting started is to set aside the time and do something, even if it is easy and doesn't seem like you are burning many calories doing it. (No, put the Doritos down and get off the couch.) I mean exercise something that involves movement of something other than your jaw. Don't worry about how hard you're working at first. Do something that is very easy for you. Just take a leisurely walk. There's nothing very demanding about that. Establish the habit of setting aside time to exercise first. You can worry about performance and calories burned later.

When you are extremely overweight, you don't feel good. You are tired most of the time. When you're sitting there like a lump on your couch, it seems that the exercise will just make you more tired. Actually, the opposite is true. Stand up right now. Take three deep breaths, holding each one for about 30 seconds and letting it out slowly. Now, run in place for about 30 seconds. Don't you feel better? Do this now, otherwise you'll have no idea what I'm talking about.

You've just increased the rate your blood circulates, that's obvious. What's not as obvious is that you've also increased the rate your lymphatic system circulates. The increased circulation of blood brings more oxygen to your tissues. The increase in lymphatic drainage removes waste that surrounds your cells. Sending oxygen to your cells and removing the wastes through exercise make you feel better even when you only do it for a few minutes. If you exercise every day, you'll feel better all the time. Of course, if you are extremely overweight, have a heart condition or any other health problems, you should consult a physician before exercising.

The worst case scenario is that you are in terrible shape and extremely obese. It may take eight or ten weeks of pre-exercise before you can concentrate on doing much of a workout. Start by taking slow walks, then little by little, increase your walking speed for short periods of time, then for longer periods until the entire walk is a brisk one. Don't push yourself too hard. If the exercise is too hard, you won't do it.

⊏⊐ *Even if you weigh more than a small country, have to stay away from the beach because you influence the tides and wish to God that you were only 45 pounds overweight, it is important that you set aside the time and perform some activity of which you are capable. Even if it seems as if you're doing very little, set aside the time and do something. As you become healthier you can increase the amount of activity. Ideally you should set aside 30 minutes per day every day.*

Take Your Pulse As You Exercise

It is important that the exercise is not painful or seems as if it is an overwhelming amount of work. The best way to tell if you're doing an appropriate amount of work is to take your pulse at some point during the activity. You can take your pulse at the radial or the carotid arteries.

The bone of the forearm that is on the same side as the thumb is called the radius. The radial pulse is found just inside (medial to) the radius, near where the wrist bends.

The carotid pulse is found on either side of the windpipe. The carotid pulse is a little stronger and will be easier for you to find than the radial pulse. If you still can't find your pulse, jump up and down a few times and try again. Now just count the number of times it beats for one minute. If you're lazy, like I am, just count the number of beats in 15 seconds and multiply by four.

Your Ideal Pulse Rate During Exercise

During exercise you want your heart rate to be between 70 percent and 90 percent of your maximum heart rate. Roughly, your maximum heart rate is 220 minus your age. The chart below shows what your ideal heart rate should be during exercise.

Age	Pulse Range
20	140 — 180
30	133 — 171
40	126 — 162
50	119 — 153
60	112 — 144
70	105 — 135

If you are really out of shape or extremely overweight, you'll find that it doesn't take a lot of activity to reach your target heart rate. If you're really heavy — the kind of heavy where you have to memorize what color shoes you have on — a walk around the block may make you reach your target heart rate. That's fine. Start your exercise program by walking for 30 minutes a day. Do it every day and remember to check your pulse. As your cardiovascular system improves, you'll have to move faster to get your heart rate up.

Working at your target heart rate is considered moderate exercise, during which approximately half of the calories burned come from carbohydrates (blood sugar and glycogen) and the other half come from fat. Moderate exercise is strenuous enough to improve your cardiovascular system without having to spend a long time exercising to derive any benefit.

There are several reasons to work out at your target heart rate. Primarily it is an efficient way to increase cardiovascular fitness. In practical terms, this means that as time passes you will feel better and be able to do more. Also exercising at your target heart rate is reasonably comfortable. You should be able to converse normally while exercising. It will be easy for you to stay on an exercise program if you're not choking and wheezing, trying to keep up with Jane Fonda.

Common Exercise Errors

There are two common mistakes you can make when planning an exercise program. One is to overdo it and become discouraged or possibly injured while attempting to exercise at a level that your body is not ready for. Don't try to keep up with people who are in better shape than you are and don't follow any exercise videos or classes that are too difficult.

The second mistake is to decide on a level of exercise that is too easy. If you do not check your heart rate and increase your level of exercise as your physical fitness improves, you may plateau. Your weight loss may slow down or stop. You need to let your heart (rate) be your guide. Checking your pulse will keep you from overdoing it in the beginning and will keep you from underexercising later.

As time goes on, your activity will need to be more strenuous in order to enable you to reach your target heart rate. It is important for you to continue to increase the pace and amount of exercise you do. You will become more energetic and your health will improve, which is what your goal really should be. Think of thinness as a nice side effect.

How Frequently Should You Exercise?

You should exercise *every day*. You are better off exercising moderately every day than doing a hard workout every two or three days. If you prefer to have a strenuous workout every two or three days, that's fine. It's even advisable to have a few days in the week when you work out harder than the minimum. Just do a short 15- or 20-minute workout on your days off. Exercising consistently every day, rather than every two or three days, will do much more to increase your resting metabolism and decrease your appetite.

You Are An Athlete

Think of yourself as an athlete. You need to apply the principles of athletic training to your exercise program. Start at a certain level and keep increasing. Make it your goal to become increasingly fit. I realize that every time you see an exercise video, go to a gym or watch a syndicated exercise program on TV, the people working out don't look as if they need to lose weight. All of the sports training books and videos seem to be geared to people who don't seem to have that far to go to become fit. Don't become discouraged. Remember, you are on your way to becoming that fit. Think of yourself as an athlete, even if you're 100 pounds overweight. Walking that extra 100 pounds around the block is quite an athletic feat. Give a skinny person a 100-pound bag of cement to carry around the block, and he'll get tired too. The heavier you are, the more work (calories burned) it takes to do the same activity as a thin person. If you weigh 100 pounds (unlikely if you've bought this book — unless you're two and a half feet tall), you burn four calories per minute walking on pavement. If you weigh 220 pounds, you burn about eight calories per minute walking.

Realistic Expectations

Don't expect too much of yourself, especially at first. The amount you exercise should be determined by your own body and what it is capable of doing. You see people on TV or in gyms doing physical activity that absolutely seems impossible to you. Gyms may seem intimidating because everyone else seems to be in such good shape. Don't worry about it. Everyone is too worried about how big their pecs are getting or what the girl across the gym has on under her tight leotard to worry about you. After a couple of visits you'll feel right at home, wondering if the girl in the tight leotard or the guy with the big pecs has on a wedding ring. If you don't know where to begin, just find an activity that appeals to you and start doing it. Take your pulse to make sure you're working at an appropriate pace.

For some reason everyone seems to be hung up on jogging or running. If you're fat and your knees hurt, jogging is unthinkable (and it should be). High-impact exercise, such as running and jogging are not advisable. Running is popular because it burns a lot of calories and is good for muscle tone and cardiovascular fitness, but there are more injuries associated with running than with many other exercises.

There are other problems associated with jogging. I started to jog, but the department of streets and sanitation complained because the road repair crews had to work overtime. High-impact exercises are not good for anyone's feet, ankles or knees, let alone someone who is overweight and out of shape. Stay away from high-impact aerobics. A nicely built woman in a tight leotard bouncing around is good marketing, but not good exercise. It may get your heart rate up, but you might get hurt.

Avoiding Injury

One of the worst things that can happen is to become excited and motivated about getting in shape, only to be sidelined by an injury that could have been avoided. Power walking is better than running. Low-impact is better than high-impact aerobics. Your lower back, hips, knees, ankles and feet will thank you.

If you are not accustomed to exercising, it will be very easy to injure yourself. This is especially true if you've exercised in the past, but haven't done so for a while. Try not to exercise as rigorously as you did five or ten years ago. You're older and fatter now, and you'll probably hurt yourself.

You should also do a warm-up and a cool-down. Basically, it's just doing your exercise at an easy level at the beginning and at the end of your workout. For instance, if you use an exercycle, turn down the tension and just pedal slowly for five minutes at the beginning and at the end of the exercise session.

Spend some time stretching before you exercise — especially stretch areas that will be doing the most work. There's a book by Bob Anderson called *Stretching* (catchy title, easy to remember). It's a good book. It'll show you what areas of your body to stretch for the type of exercise that you're doing. It has good illustrations and it shows you the proper positioning and intensity of the stretch. New research indicates that stretching may not be as necessary to the prevention of injury as previously thought, but there's nothing conclusive yet. Stretch before exercising anyway. Flexibility is part of good health.

What Exercise Is Right For You?

Different types of exercise burn calories at different rates. The more large muscles you use, the faster you will burn calories. For instance, cross-country skiing burns up more calories than bicycling. It is a more efficient exercise — you use upper body muscles as well as lower body muscles cross-country skiing. You also burn more calories because the exercise is weight-bearing (standing instead of sitting).

I bought an exercycle with handles that move to exercise the upper body. It offers the same upper and lower body movement as cross-country skiing, but the calories are not burned as quickly on the bike because fewer calories are burned sitting than are burned standing.

If you purchase an exercise machine, how efficient it is may not matter much at first. A machine that exercises the muscles of your upper and lower body may be too hard for you in the beginning. The more muscles you use during an exercise, the more calories per hour you'll burn. But that also means more work. If you're out of shape, exercising on an efficient machine (such as a Nordic Track) may be too intense. Your heart may be working so hard that you'll hardly be able to stand up, let alone converse. Later, when you become more physically fit, an efficient machine is nice to have because you can lose more weight in less time.

Interval Training

I have a relative in his sixties who hadn't exercised in a long time. He bought a Nordic Track. After two minutes of exercise, his pulse shot up. He had to lie on the bed for a while, gasping for breath. If you've never been on a Nordic Track, it's hard to do it slowly. It's an excellent machine, but you almost have to be already in shape to use it. He couldn't pace himself. Having invested $750 in the thing, he was determined to use it. He worked out for a minute at a time, which kept him safely at the pre-gasp-and-choke level and would repeat this several times a day. Now he's in good enough shape to use the machine regularly. If you're able to use one, the Nordic Track is great. They are well made and you can burn a lot of calories in a short amount of time, but many people complain that they'd have to get in shape before they could use one.

His workout was an example of interval training. When an athlete does interval training, he or she will work at full intensity for a predetermined amount of time, rest for approximately three times the amount of time of the workout, then repeat the work-rest sequence (e.g., work for one minute, rest for three). The advantage here is that the athlete can work at high intensity for a relatively long period of time. Examples of this are circuit weight training and some of the settings on the Life-cycle. Keep in mind that this *may* be a strain on the heart of a sedentary individual. *Again, check with your doctor before beginning any exercise program.* Continuous training at your target heart rate will serve you just fine.

Make Up Your Own Exercise Program

To develop your own exercise program you don't need special equipment or even a health club. You can do 15 minutes of a stationary brisk march. (Thirty minutes is better, but if time is an issue for you, make sure you exercise at least 15 minutes per day.) If you have a hard time reaching your target heart rate, you can exaggerate the movement of your arms and legs or step on a milk crate or foot stool every other step.

You could choreograph your own aerobics program. Begin by stretching. Reach very high into the air with your left arm and lean to the right. Feel the muscles on your side stretch for about 30 seconds. (Always hold a stretch for at least 30 seconds and don't bounce.) Do the same thing leaning to the left. Turn to the right and lunge like a fencer. Keep your right leg in front of you, bent, and your left leg behind you, straight. Feel the stretch in the front of the left leg. Hold it for 30 seconds.

Do the other side. Use a brisk march as your basic movement. Use a milk crate or a foot stool to step up on. Add other movements to the march, such as touching your elbow to your opposite knee, touching your hand to the opposite foot behind you, doing exaggerated arm movements such as punching at the sky and exaggerating the leg movements. Let your pulse determine how hard you work. It should be no problem to find 15 minutes a day to do this (preferably 30 minutes). Even if you work a lot of hours or if you travel, you should be able to find time to do this. If you watch any TV at all, you have no excuse. If turning off the TV is too much for you to bear, then purchase a closed-captioning device and do it while you watch the tube.

Ideally there should be no homolateral movements in the exercise. A homolateral movement is when the same arm and leg go in the same direction. An example of this is a jumping jack (which you should avoid anyway because of the high impact). The right arm goes to the side the same time as the right leg, as does the left arm and leg. Neurologically this is not a good idea. The human body is designed for walking. When you walk, your left arm goes forward at the same time your right leg goes forward. This is called the cross-crawl pattern and it is better for your neurological organization if your exercise program respects that. When choosing a video program or a machine, make sure you can warm up adequately, avoid high-impact and homolateral movements and always remember to cool down. Also make sure you can do the exercise and stay at your target heart rate.

Choosing Exercise Equipment

If you decide to buy an exercise machine, the type you buy is not as important as the quality of the product. Pick an exercise that you're likely to do, whether it's rowing, bicycling or cross-country skiing. Spend the money to get something that is well-made. If the parts on inferior equipment become loose, the machines won't work smoothly. Cheap exercycles begin to wobble and pedal unevenly after a while. Unfortunately you get what you pay for. If the equipment doesn't work well, you won't use it. A $59.95 cross-country ski machine will sit in the corner collecting dust. If money is an issue for you, do calisthenics or walk. A poorly made exercise machine is just wasted money.

Overcoming Boredom

One of the major problems with exercise is boredom, especially if you're just sitting on a rowing machine or exercycle counting the minutes before you can get off the damned thing. You should take some steps to make your exercise more enjoyable. One way is to select music that really makes you feel good and play it during your workout.

I like to listen to rock and roll when I exercise. It's energetic. During my workout, I listen to a Dire Straits tape that my wife and I often listened to when we were first dating. Pick music that brings back good memories or means something to you. It will put you in a good mood and make the time go by faster. Whether you like jazz, rock, classical or, God help you, disco, the music will make the right hemisphere of your brain more involved with the activity than the left hemisphere.

Your right hemisphere is the spacially oriented, intuitive, creative part of your brain. The left hemisphere is the linear, logical part of your brain. When you're on the exercycle, your left hemisphere is thinking, "God! This is boring, only 17 minutes to go. Losing another pound is just like taking a cup of sand out of the Sahara Desert, so why should I bother?" "I'm too fat; this is stupid," "My butt hurts."

If you play music, your right hemisphere will be replaying images of you and Betty Lou (or Billy Bob) groping in the back seat of your father's Buick, as you did when that song was popular. The right hemisphere of your brain will be imagining what it would be like to play an instrument as well as the musicians performing the music. It will allow you to get lost in the music and maybe even play a little mental air guitar. When exercising, listen to the music and let the right side of your brain take over. Time will pass quickly and you may even enjoy yourself. You can even try rap:

> Yeah I'm the one who got too fat.
> I thought that Twinkies were where it was at
> I'm here to tell you I'm gettin' lean
> But if I miss a meal I get too mean
> So I chain myself to an exercise machine . . .

Another way to counteract boredom is to vary your exercises. The more kinds of exercise you have to do, the more likely you'll work out regularly. One of the advantages of going to a health club is the variety of equipment and classes available. You could do a different type of workout each day. If you're doing the same exercise at home every day, going to a health club is a great way to break the monotony a few days a week. At a club there's usually some kind of upbeat music playing, there's a lot to see (including attractive members of the opposite sex). It's a more interesting place to work out (very pleasing to the right hemisphere of your brain) than home and, unlike at home, there is no temptation to turn on "Wheel of Fortune" and forget the whole thing.

Exercising At Home Or At A Club

I belong to a club that has good facilities and is reasonably priced. (I won't tell you the name, but Cher recommends it.) I don't know if I'd have joined it if my schedule didn't allow me to exercise during the midmorning hours. The club gets very busy in the late afternoon because the owners tend to oversell the facility. You often have to wait for the piece of equipment you want to use. It seems as if everyone wants to look like Cher (including a lot of the men here on the near-north side of town).

The Stair-Master is particularly popular. People often wait in line for it, three-deep, usually after taking the elevator to get to the club. (It's on the seventh floor.) If you'll be working out in the evening, go to the club at that time and see how busy it gets before you purchase a membership. If you can discipline yourself to go in the morning, most places are not busy.

Even if you join a health club and go regularly, make arrangements to be able to do some sort of exercise at home as well. Weather, traffic, changes in your schedule and other disruptions can keep you from going. If you miss exercising for a few days in a row, starting again becomes very difficult. Have something to fall back on at home.

At home I have my exercycle and some video tapes I've made from exercise shows on TV. "The Body Electric" is pretty good for muscle toning. There's another show on cable that's also pretty good. It's taught by a husband and wife team. I try to watch it when the wife teaches (not for the reason you're thinking). She tends to do less jumping around and her instructions are clearer. He's not bad, but when he gets everyone jumping or running in place, I usually go into a brisk march. Initially I tried to do the high-impact exercise, but the downstairs neighbors complained about the plaster on their ceiling cracking. (We're expecting some engineers to come out and check the building for structural damage.)

I don't mention these shows to tell you to follow them. When I first started exercising, I physically couldn't keep up with either of them. The point is to vary your exercise to keep it interesting. Enjoy yourself when you exercise. The more you enjoy exercising, the more you'll do and the easier it will be for you to lose weight.

The Payoff

The most difficult part of exercising is getting started. The more weight you have to lose, the more futile it will seem, which is why it's important to enjoy the process. Exercise moderately, vary your activity and listen to music. Then exercise just might become pleasant for you. Weight loss is not the only benefit of exercise. As your cardiovascular system improves, you will have more energy. You will feel better in general very soon after you start. Exercise is its own reward. If you approach it correctly, you will enjoy exercising for its own sake.

Make Yourself Work Harder

Take the stairs instead of the elevator. If you work at the top of the Sears Tower, you can reach your target weight in about two days. Seriously, find ways to become more active throughout the day. If you take a bus to work, get off a couple of blocks before and walk the rest of the way. Ten minutes of walking, which replaces ten minutes of sitting, means that you are burning an extra 48 calories. In a year that amounts to about 18,000 calories which is about five pounds of fat.

Get a bicycle and use it for some of your errands. You will burn between five and eight calories per minute. Ride it to work if that is possible.

Exercise doesn't have to be in concentrated doses in order to burn calories. You burn calories doing any activity. If you go ten miles, you burn the same number of calories whether you walk or run. You are moving the same amount of weight the same distance. It takes the same amount of energy, regardless of the speed. The difference between walking and running ten miles lies in the amount of time, not in the amount of energy spent. You can run ten miles in under an hour. Walking would take you two hours or better. The same number of calories are burned either way.

You might be thinking, "Why do I have to exercise? Why don't I just do a little more walking?" I hope you're not thinking that, but you might be. The workout sessions will help you to:

- Lose weight quickly
- Increase your metabolism
- Improve your cardiovascular fitness
- Give you more energy.

Don't try to eliminate the exercise.

When primitive man saw a saber-toothed tiger, he didn't say, "I'm pretty active, I don't need the exercise." He ran like hell! If he had to forage for food, he didn't say, "I already ran today when I saw that tiger. I don't need any extra activity." He still had to walk around and find his nuts and berries. He couldn't call Domino's Nut and Berry and have them delivered with a video. Our society has made us sedentary.

You need to be active.

Destroy Your Television

That may be a little extreme. Just give it to someone you don't like.

Try to cut down on your television viewing. A 180-pound person burns about 1.7 calories per minute watching TV. (You're always burning calories, unless you're dead — watching TV is as close as you can come to that.) Compare that to walking, which burns 6.5 calories per minute for the same size person. That's a little over 105,000 calories per year if you replace an hour of television with a one-hour walk. That represents a loss of 30 pounds of fat at the end of a year.

TV is a time trap. It's not uncommon for patients to tell me that they don't have time to prepare proper meals or to exercise, but they always manage to find time to catch the "Gomer Pyle" reruns.

The television also programs you to eat junk, "Aren't you hungry?" "Nothing says lovin' like somethin' from the oven." "The taste of a whole new generation." "Make a run for the border." "Betcha can't eat just one." How do you spell relief? T-U-R-N-I-T-O-F-F!

If commercials weren't effective, companies wouldn't spend millions of dollars on them. If that kind of programming went toward urging you to eat right, you wouldn't need this book.

I'm vain enough to think that commercials don't affect me and that no one can program me. The following quotation is from Jay Conrad Levinson in his book, *Guerilla Marketing Attack:*

En route from JFK Airport in the taxi, we talked about the up-coming meeting. The driver, overhearing our conversation, leaned back and asked, "You guys in the ad game?"

"Yes," we told him.

"You guys really believe that crap works?" he asked, and he earnestly wanted an answer.

"Sure we do," one of us said. "We wouldn't be having this meeting if we didn't."

The cab driver set us straight:

"Well, I sure as hell don't believe it works. I can tell you this — I've never bought anything because of advertising and I never will."

"What kind of toothpaste do you use?" one of us asked.

"Well, I brush with Gleem," he told us. "But it's in no way connected with the advertising. It's because I drive a cab and I really can't brush after every meal."

That's a funny story, and true, based on Gleem's marketing theme at the time: "For people who can't brush after every meal." But it's not that funny when you consider how many products you've bought because of some aspect of the marketing. You won't be able to identify many. But if you go through your refrigerator, food cabinets, clothes closets, and medicine chest, and think of your appliances, car and whatnot, you'll be a bit shocked at how much marketing has motivated you. You're not unique in this respect: It's the same way with almost everyone. That's why so much time passes before most marketing works. Accessing the unconscious mind of a human being is not all that easy.

Just because you hear that Pizza Hut is "makin' it great" and don't rush out to buy a pizza doesn't mean the commercial doesn't have an effect on you. The effect is more subtle than that. One day your blood sugar will get a little low and you'll get hungry. Pizza will flash in your mind. Suddenly you're not just hungry, you're hungry for pizza, cookies, burgers, fries, donuts or whatever junk food has been planted in your subconcious. The junk food commercials usually plant pretty vivid images that are recalled later. "Doesn't work on me, but you know, every once in a while I just have to have a greasy hamburger." Sound familiar?

This is another reason you have to spend time visualizing and programming yourself to want to eat right. If you don't program yourself, a fast-food chain will gladly do it.

I don't really expect you to give up television. I can't imagine Monday nights without "Murphy Brown" (with football during the commercials), but limit your viewing to things you really want to see.

☐══════ *Don't vegetate in front of the set just because there's nothing else to do.* Stop watching the commercials, *especially food commercials. Go into another room, get a remote to change channels or get up and change channels yourself during the commercials.*

Get Busy, Stop Being Sedentary

Regular aerobic exercise should be part of your routine. You should also walk more and use elevators and cars less. There is one more thing you can do to increase your activity level.

Play

So far we've only discussed activity as a discipline but it doesn't have to be all work. There are lots of sports and other activities that are fun and educational. If you watch a lot of television or sit around during your free time, develop other interests and activities that are not sedentary.

You've already seen the difference walking an extra hour every day can make. The same principle applies to other activities. Golf nine or 18 holes once a week (don't use the cart). Play with your kids. Put a basketball hoop in the backyard or get a ping-pong table. Practice yoga. Have sex. (It varies, but you can burn about seven calories per minute, more with a partner. I find it a great way to burn an extra 10 or 12 calories.) Get interested in something new that keeps you active. Learn to dance the Lambada, take fencing lessons, start a garden, go bowling or take up mountain climbing.

If you are extremely overweight, you probably can't imagine doing more than your day already demands of you. Trust me, you're going to start feeling better and have more energy. Use that extra energy to enjoy yourself and to get some extra results. Our prehistoric ancestors were active all day long. They didn't sit at a desk or spend their days in front of a computer terminal. You need to find ways to be more active, especially if you have a sedentary job.

I know what you're thinking, "When I get home, I'm tired. I don't have enough energy to do much more than sit in front of the TV." That's probably true, but if you do some deep breathing for a couple of minutes and spend a few minutes on the exercycle, you'll be in a whole different frame of mind. Don't make any decisions about the evening until you've done this. You will have more energy and will be more able to be active. This is especially true if you are usually sedentary.

━━━ *Our sedentary free time is when most of us absent-mindedly eat. Most of my patients trying to lose weight tell me they have great willpower during the day but at night they tend to overeat. If you're just sitting around, it's very easy to want to eat. You can kill two birds with one stone: burn calories while being active and keep yourself from thinking about food at the same time.*

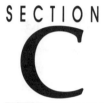

Controlling
What You Eat

ontrolling what you eat is more important than controlling how much you eat. The quality of the food
you eat is much more important than the quantity. If the food you
eat is full of empty calories, you will tend to eat more of it. Eating
whole foods in their natural state will satisfy your appetite, eating
refined foods will increase it. It is useless to try to control how
much you eat until you are in control of what you eat.

Many of the things in this chapter could also fit into the next
chapter: "Limiting Calories." Many of the foods that cause you to
overeat are high in calories. Giving up sugar and fried foods will
help to decrease your appetite and put you in control of what you
eat. They are also high-calorie foods and giving them up will
decrease your caloric intake. They are listed in this section because the number of calories in a Coke or a dish of French fries
are secondary to what "food" such as this does to your ability to
control your eating.

Don't Diet Or Get Hung Up On Calories

Be more concerned with the quality of the food you're eating than its caloric content. Two powdered donuts have about 228 calories. A bowl of split pea soup with two slices of whole wheat bread has 238 calories. Guess which ends up on your hips. The donuts don't have much nutritional value, so it's likely that you'll be hungry a little while after eating them (probably for more sugar). The soup and bread will be more satisfying and you won't become hungry again as quickly.

Dieting is unpleasant and reducing calories makes most people feel deprived and hungry. It doesn't matter how you package the reduction. You can get a set of cards that tell you what to eat. You can get packaged food sold to you in conjunction with counseling or you can drink protein powder, but the results are always the same: If you don't get enough food, you'll make up for it later. Dieting simply doesn't work.

Ketogenic Diets Are Dangerous

Dieting is so unpleasant that the public has been sold some screwy programs that promised to either speed up the process or allow them to "lose weight without being hungry." Ketogenic diets seem to fill these criteria.

Ketogenic refers to the waste product formed when fat breaks down. Normally the body uses carbohydrates as fuel. A ketogenic diet is very low in carbohydrates, so the body is forced to burn fat for fuel. These diets were popular for a while because they allowed the dieter to eat all that he or she wanted, as long as it wasn't carbohydrates.

I went to school with a student who was a little over-weight, about 20 or 25 pounds. One day I noticed that he was a lot thinner, close to what he should weigh. I commented to him about how quickly he had lost the weight. It was as if he left his spare tire home one morning. He was very pleased to hear my comment. He said that he started this great new diet a few weeks ago that turned his body "into a fat-burning machine." He could eat as much as he wanted and still lose weight. The trick was that he couldn't have any carbohydrates in his diet. I saw him eat six eggs and nothing else for breakfast one morning.

This is a pretty dangerous program. There's risk of kidney or heart damage. Many essential nutrients are not provided. To a person who has just lost 20 pounds it may seem to be worth the risk: It isn't. When we graduated, he was at least ten pounds heavier than he was when he started the diet.

Other ketogenic diets are the Atkins diet, the drinking man's diet (these are high-fat, low-carbohydrate diets) and the Pennington diet (high protein, low carbohydrate). These diets came into existence because losing weight by counting calories was too slow and too unpleasant. Medically supervised fasts are also ketogenic. This is basically controlled starvation and very dangerous, which is why these programs must be done under a doctor's supervision.

Low-Fat Diets

Things have gone full circle now. Carbohydrates, which used to be avoided in weight loss programs, are now being hailed as "heart smart" foods. In the eighties and now in the nineties the way to lose weight is by avoiding fats.

The Pritikin diet is the most popular of these. On Pritikin's program the dieter eats fewer than 10 percent of his or her calories as fat. The program has merit in our modern industrialized society. For one thing, fats are, well, fattening. They are very high in calories, more so than proteins and carbohydrates. Animal fats have been implicated in heart disease and cancer and, because of this, we have taken the attitude that all fats are bad.

One of the major problems with animal fat is that environmental pollution is stored in animal fat, not to mention the hormones, antibiotics and other drugs fed to animals by the food producer. It makes vegetarianism an attractive life-style.

Even the vegetable oils we buy today are not what they were a hundred years ago. They are extracted by heat or chemicals and are, at best, empty calories and, at worst, toxic.

There are two problems with Pritikin's program. It is hard to stay on. In fact, it would be much easier to become a vegetarian than to stay on the Pritikin diet. If you're worried about cholesterol, a vegan, the most extreme vegetarian, consumes no cholesterol. The other problem is that you need some fat in order to get essential fatty acids and oil soluble vitamins.

You need to distinguish between good fat and bad fat. Natural oils, present in legumes and whole grains, are high in many nutrients we need. Eggs are very high in vitamin A and essential fatty acids. (Eggs from chickens that are allowed to roam free and that are fed grains rather than man-made feed are high in these nutrients.) Vegetable oils are good for you, if they are not extracted by heat or chemicals or stored in the light. Be less concerned about what the oil is extracted from and more concerned about how it was extracted. You should also avoid fried foods and hydrogenated fats. A good book to read on this subject is, *Fats And Oils* by Udo Erasmus.

Even though nuts and avocados are "high fat" foods, they need not be avoided. Legumes and whole grains should be eaten often. (For what it's worth, they are "cholesterol-free" — as are all vegetables, since cholesterol is only found in animal products.) You may find that eating raw nuts or avocados will keep you from craving greasy burgers, fried foods, mayonnaise or other high-fat foods.

It is true that as a society we eat too much meat and dairy, and we would be healthier if we obtained our fats and proteins from vegetable sources. But if you are not ready to give up these foods, don't worry about it. Concentrate instead on the quality of your food.

While Pritikin's program may be good as a last-ditch effort for someone with cholesterol levels out in the stratosphere, it is not a good program for the general population. It probably is no more beneficial than simple vegetarianism, even though it is a harder program to adhere to.

Dieting Cycles Are Futile

There is a cycle to dieting. You've seen people go through this or maybe you've gone through it yourself. First there's the discovery of a new diet. Perhaps one or more of your friends have gone from a size 18 to a size five or you see someone on a daytime talk show who has just lost 438 pounds just in time for swimsuit season on this great new diet. So you try it.

There's the ritual of getting special foods or reading the book and planning your attack. You get psyched up; this time you're going to do it! Then you begin the program. Initial results are encouraging. You may even lose five or ten pounds in the first week. You don't feel bad; you're not even that hungry. The second week shows some weight loss, but not as much as the first. As you go into the third or fourth week, the weight loss becomes much less encouraging. Maybe not even a pound. You're enjoying the diet less. You go to bed with the Pizza Hut commercial playing in your head.

Often there is some kind of new stress in your life. Your BMW gets repossessed or your kid shaves his head and starts selling flowers at the airport. Suddenly the diet seems unbearable. (Sometimes you don't even need the extra stress to drive you to this point.) You go to the 7-Eleven in the middle of the night and buy out the Hostess cake display, hide in the basement (so no one knows — you'd been telling them how great this diet was and how easy it was to stay on) and eat the cakes. Soon you're back to your old eating habits. Now you feel guilty. If someone on a talk show could lose 438 pounds, why can't you lose 20?

You gain your weight back, plus a couple of extra pounds. After the diet, it seems as if you're having a hard time with even sensible, moderate control over your eating.

This is not your fault. Your own physiology is keeping you from losing weight. Even Dr. Peter's sensible plan of eating fewer calories than you burn has some built-in problems. Going on almost any diet will cause you to lose a lot of weight initially, sometimes as much as five or ten pounds. This is water weight. I forget which product has the slogan "Give us a week, and we'll take off the weight." They're right, they can help you to lose weight in the first week. It's no big accomplishment. Any program can.

When you first begin dieting, you burn up stored carbohydrates rather than fat. The carbohydrates have more water (hence the term "water weight"), and therefore weigh more than fat. Fasting for two days will give you that same quick weight loss until you start eating again.

As a diet progresses, the rate of the weight loss decreases. Your body is making an attempt to stop this alarming loss of fat. It interprets the loss of weight as starvation and tries to help you survive by slowing down your metabolism. Your body doesn't seem to understand that you have another 90 pounds to go before starvation becomes an issue.

Your metabolism slows down and your appetite increases, sometimes becoming uncontrollable. That's why sensible eating seems impossible after a diet. Many people successfully follow a diet only to fail on the maintenance portion of the program. The tendency toward binge eating after a diet is just your body's attempt to help you get that precious weight back. It has nothing to do with a lack of willpower.

Severe caloric restriction can reduce your metabolism by as much as 45%. After a few failed diets you become one of those people who says, "I don't understand it, I eat hardly anything, yet I can't lose weight. I just look at food and get fat." As your metabolism slows down you also become tired all of the time. The results of your dieting are that you are tired, overweight and still not eating enough to satisfy yourself. When you're this miserable, it's not surprising if a hot fudge sundae is the highlight of your day.

If you are overweight, you have problems with foods that are unique to you. You may have habits, cravings, digestive problems or even hidden food allergies. You have your own metabolic rate. You are a biochemically unique individual. A program that some expert picks for most of the population may not be right for you. For some reason many people love programs that tell them exactly what to eat. They seem to want to put on blinders and have someone map out a plan they can follow without thinking and lose weight. That's the appeal of programs such as the Scarsdale diet.

Learn the right way to lose weight for you. Stop putting yourself at the mercy of "experts" and learn what you need to do to lose the weight you want.

You need to change your habits permanently. In order to do that, the changes need to be gradual and reasonable. Don't do anything extreme. Just learn which habits keep you fat and change them one at a time.

Absolutely Avoid Refined Sugar

It should be obvious to you that you should not eat sugar. I can't think of any diet that encourages you to eat desserts. Believe me, if there were a way, I'd do it — and this book would sell a million copies. Stay away from chocolate, candy, cookies, donuts, soda pop, cake, ice cream, sugared cereals and all the rest. If your sweet tooth is such that your heart is sinking as you read this and you're ready to burn this book, cheer up.

Controlling Your Sweet Tooth

It is very easy to bring sugar cravings under control. Just make sure you don't go more than two hours without snacking. If lunch is at noon and dinner at six, eat a piece of fruit at two and at four. Fruit is your snack of choice because it has natural sugar and will curb your craving. If this doesn't work, try taking a little vitamin B complex. Most people are amazed how easy it is to give up sweets.

If you feel that you will miss dessert after dinner, Karen Barkie has written an excellent cook book called *Sweet And Sugar-Free*. This book is full of healthy desserts sweetened with fruit and fruit juices.

Refined Sugar Is Empty Calories

A Mars bar has 230 calories, more than 10 grams of fat and no food value. Give up empty calories and fat. You don't have to worry about the number of calories you eat if everything you eat has food value. It's the empty calories that make you fat. Instead you could have three ounces of lean flank steak, a potato and green beans for about 250 calories. Granted that's no butter for the potato and beans (add 72 for two pats), but the point is that you are consuming the same number of calories when you eat sweets as you do in a complete meal.

You can have an entire meal for just a few more calories than are in that candy bar. It's a pretty low-calorie meal, selected just to illustrate a point. A less lean cut of meat would increase the calories by 100 or more. But you're looking at a meal that will fill you up and supply you with many necessary vitamins and minerals as compared to a snack that will leave you craving more sugar in a few hours.

The Damage Sugar Does To Your Body

As bad as sugar is for you, considering the number of unnecessary calories is nothing compared to what it does to your body. Sugar will really interfere with your attempt to lose weight, not in the extra calories of a sugary snack, but by making you crave more sugar later. It gives you calories and, other than a temporary increase in blood sugar, it doesn't satisfy any of your body's nutritional needs.

There are also some other problems with eating sweets. Sweets change the pH of your digestive system. "Big deal!" you say. But it is a big deal. The enzyme systems that digest your food are pH-dependent. Also the bacteria that live in your large intestine are sensitive to changes in pH. There is a delicate balance of nature in your intestines between bacteria and yeast. If you eat a lot of sugar, you create an environment that favors yeast growth. Too much yeast can cause a lot of problems. You may tend to bloat or get tired when you eat. You may even develop allergies. Many women become prone to yeast infections.

Sugar is also hard on your endocrine system. It puts stress on the pancreas and on the adrenal glands. Eating too much sugar can make you tired all of the time. If you are tired and you eat a lot of sugar, give it up and you'll feel better.

Occasionally someone has a lot of trouble giving up sugar. It may be due to problems with digestion and absorption. Refined sugar is very easily absorbed. If a person is not digesting protein very well, he or she may tend to crave sugar. You see this a lot in older people. They don't care much for meat, but they love desserts.

As a person gets older, he or she produces less hydrochloric acid for digestion, making it more difficult to digest protein. Some think this is why people get osteoarthritis. The body needs protein to sustain life. It is needed by the brain, kidneys, heart and other vital organs. When there is a deficiency (in this case because of a problem digesting the protein), it will steal the protein from less important areas such as joint surfaces.

Joint movement is not as important as kidney, heart or brain function. The body sacrifices ease of movement, which is a luxury compared to these other functions. Such a person should take supplements to improve digestion which in turn will help bring the sweet tooth under control.

Another problem some people have is an allergy to either corn (and therefore corn syrup, one of the more common sweeteners), cane sugar or even chocolate. People who are allergic to a food tend to be addicted to it, much the same way an alcoholic is addicted. In fact, Theron Randolph (a noted allergist and a man who can be considered the founder of clinical ecology) calls alcoholism the ultimate food allergy. We will talk more about allergies later. They are a major cause of overeating and obesity.

So you can see there is a bigger problem with sugar than the obvious one of calories. That can of soda is more than an extra 150 calories. It is a can of fatigue, digestive problems and endocrine stress — a taste for a whole new generation.

Don't Starve Yourself

Not eating will not make you lose weight effectively. Skipping meals and reducing calories will give you a temporary initial weight loss, but ultimately it will slow down your metabolism. If you persist in starving yourself, your appetite will come back with a vengeance. Your body will work at holding onto its fat during what it considers to be a potentially life-threatening situation.

Ever since Dr. Peters wrote her book and introduced the concept of the calorie, we've been simplistically trying to lose weight by eating fewer calories than we burn. It simply doesn't work (at least not without exercise). Your body is more complicated than that.

If you are in the habit of skipping meals, chances are that you have a sweet tooth. In the office I seem to hear the statements, "I never eat breakfast" and "I'd rather die than give up chocolate," from the same person. If you don't eat enough during the day and your blood sugar gets low, you instinctively know that a chocolate bar will be absorbed quickly and raise your blood sugar. The sugar seems to give you a lift, which makes you crave it. Even after you've eaten an entire meal late in the day, the desire for sugar lingers. You may find yourself eating dessert late at night after you've eaten plenty for dinner.

The problem with using sweets to raise your blood sugar is that it raises the blood sugar suddenly, making your pancreas work hard to produce insulin so the body can get the sugar into the cells. A lot of times you produce more insulin than you need, so later your subconscious says to you, "Gee, I need a little more sugar to go with this insulin." So in a couple of hours you want something else that's sweet. If you have more sugar, you will probably overproduce insulin, making you want more sugar later and so on throughout the day.

⊏══⊐ *Eating regular meals is one way to curb a sweet tooth. If you starve yourself, you may find yourself eating more sugar than you want. Even if you don't end up craving sugar, skipping meals will only slow down your metabolism and thwart any weight loss. Eventually it may lead to binge eating.*

Eat If You're Hungry

Sometimes you've just eaten, but you want to snack. That's okay, just don't eat junk food. Distinguish between genuine hunger and nervous eating. If you absentmindedly eat, notice yourself eating without realizing it or watch yourself craving the same foods all of the time, that's another problem. But sometimes if you didn't get enough food at your last meal or your blood sugar is a little low and you're hungry, then eat. Snack on fresh fruit or vegetables. They will stop you from being hungry and won't add many calories to your diet. It is important that you don't ignore your hunger; you'll only end up eating something worse later.

If you're hungry all of the time or you can't seem to get full, you may have problems with digestion or have food allergies. Those topics will be covered later.

If you're used to dieting, you're not being permitted to eat beyond the parameters of the diet. On most diets you'll be hungry at least some of the time. Even diets that permit you to eat unlimited amounts of food are still limited in their selection, so you don't get to eat what you're hungry for. On an all-protein diet, it's surprising how unsatisfying your eighth egg of the day or your fourth steak is when you haven't had any carbohydrates.

This isn't a diet. Snack all you want to but limit your snacks to fresh fruits and vegetables. If you're hungry and you've been eating regular meals, an apple and a large glass of water will fill you up. An apple only has about 80 calories.

If you have a sweet tooth, it is especially important that you snack, even to the point of anticipating your hunger. Usually that's enough to keep you from craving sugar and desserts. You could eat every two hours; it may even be necessary. Snacking during the day won't cause you to eat more food than you now consume, in fact, it may even reduce your total food consumption by allowing you to keep your hunger under control.

You make your worst nutritional decisions when you are hungry, as when you skip breakfast and get to lunch a little late or, worse, skip breakfast and lunch because you are trying to lose weight. Satisfy your hunger early, when you are able to plan better for a healthy snack. If you try to ignore your hunger, you'll find that you give in to it when you're at a hot dog stand or an ice cream parlor.

Eat Whole Grains

Because of our paranoia about fat, pasta is now being lauded as a health food because it is low in fat. But most pasta is made with refined white flour, which isn't really good for you. As far as pasta being a diet food, it is mostly carbohydrates (the same stuff we avoided like the plague on the ketogenic diets). If you eat more carbohydrates than your body can burn, your body turns them into fat anyway. You can't lose weight by loading up on pasta.

There are similar problems with eating refined white flour products as there are with eating sugar. Refined white flour products are very quickly broken down and absorbed, much like sugar. They also cause the same changes in bowel pH as sugar does.

In nature, anything that contains complex carbohydrates also contains some vitamin B, vitamin E and fiber. Interestingly, B vitamins aid in carbohydrate metabolism and fiber slows down its absorption. So when you eat a whole grain, you're automatically getting the vitamins your body needs to metabolize the carbohydrates in the grain. You also get fiber into your diet.

Why Fiber Is Good

Fiber is cellulose from the cell walls of plants. You cannot digest and absorb it. Other nutrients adhere to fiber. It sort of makes your meal timed-release. Whole grain is absorbed much more slowly than enriched white flour and is not nearly as much of the burden on your pancreas. Fiber also cuts down on the number of calories and fat you absorb. It makes your bowel healthy and reduces your chances of getting cancer by increasing bowel motility and reducing the toxicity of the bowel.

Let's go back to our cave people since you have their physiology. Refined sugar and carbohydrates did not exist for them. There was nothing that had carbohydrates in it that did not also have fiber. Anytime they ate carbohydrates, they were absorbed slowly (time-released, if you will). White flour and sugar are absorbed more quickly than anything our prehistoric ancestors had. They make the pancreas produce insulin at a very rapid rate. Often the pancreas overproduces insulin and causes a hypoglycemic state. You end up with all that extra insulin and nothing for it to do except lower the blood sugar, making you become hungry or crave sweets.

"You know, it seems as if we just ate a big meal and I'm hungry again" or "I'd like something sweet." Have you ever said that? Stop eating the refined sugar and white flour products and this won't be a problem.

The Problem With Enriched Foods

Americans eat a lot of "enriched" foods. Enriching consists of removing all of the fiber, vitamins and minerals from a grain. The manufacturer then adds thiamine, riboflavin, iron calcium (a particularly popular item lately) or whatever is popular or cheap. The product is then labeled "enriched" (a wonderful example of doublespeak), implying that the manufacturer has somehow improved on nature.

You need to eat foods the way nature created them. There is a good deal of misinformation circulating out there about nutrition. We think in terms of RDAs and absolute amounts of nutrients. Most vitamins were discovered in the 1930s when our chemical know-how wasn't very sophisticated. For example, as far as the government is concerned, ascorbic acid is vitamin C, but a food that is high in vitamin C has much more in it than just ascorbic acid. Food containing vitamin C complex has bioflavenoids, vitamin K and other nutrients. Eating food that is high in vitamin C is different from taking ascorbic acid.

B complex is present in foods that contain complex carbohydrates. The B vitamins in food containing complex carbohydrates also exist in very definite proportions to each other and to certain synergistic minerals that enable them to be absorbed by your body. These important combinations are never taken into consideration when manufacturers "enrich" their products.

The chemistry of the living cell and the human body is much more complex than the chemistry that takes place in a lab or in a beaker. Biomolecules work like little factories or fine machinery. You can give a chemist a Rolex watch and he or she can analyze it and tell you how much gold, glass, quartz and other materials are in it. You can take the same watch and smash it with a hammer and, from the chemist's point of view, nothing has changed. Cellulose and starch have the same chemical formula. Chemically, there is no difference between wood and a potato, except how the molecule is arranged. Many things added to foods, put there by the manufacturers as nutrients, are as useful to the body as wood.

Natural Foods Are Better

Each cell in your body is like a little factory producing products and eliminating waste. The cells work chemically and there is an interplay between enzymes and cofactors (molecules that make the enzyme work, sort of like an ignition key in a car). There is a delicate balance in the way the body works. You have to keep this in mind when taking supplements.

Zinc is very popular right now, but there is a balance between zinc, iron and copper. If you load up the system with zinc, you upset this balance.

You should get your vitamins and minerals from food. The food should be as close to the way that nature created it as possible. That way you'll be getting good nutrition in ways that chemists haven't discovered yet. This is not to say that supplements are never necessary, but you will be less likely to need them if you are eating whole foods.

Whole grains taste better, they fill you up faster and they're better for you than refined grains. Brown rice is a wonderful food. It's loaded with minerals and vitamins, and it has taste. Ever taste plain white rice without butter, sauces or salt? It's just starch and it tastes like spackling compound. (It has about the same food value as spackling compound, too.) Ever notice how you can practically eat an entire loaf of French bread in a single sitting? You can't do that with a good whole grain bread. Perhaps whole wheat bread doesn't trigger the emotional response for you that French bread does, but you have to understand that taste preference is learned.

If you eat slowly and take time to taste your food, the natural foods end up tasting better than the refined ones.

Don't Get Hung Up On Nutritional Fads And Buzz Words

Fat And Cholesterol

We Americans are prone to dietary extremes. We eat too many fats and refined carbohydrates. Studies show a tenuous relationship between fat consumption and heart disease and suddenly the entire population is afraid of fat as if it were a deadly poison. I saw a patient the other day and suggested that he eat avocado because it was high in a nutrient that he needed. He waved a cross made of chicken bones in the air, reached into a little leather bag he had and threw some kind of dust in my face, then shouted in horror, "Avocados are high in fat!" as he gestured rhythmically and ordered the evil spirit to be gone.

We are currently in a backlash against the high-fat diet. People are afraid of high blood pressure and heart disease, and rightfully so. Eating a diet that consists of 40 percent fat is not a good idea but it doesn't mean that fat is poison. It is a lot like staying away from water because you know that people have drowned in it. The truth of the matter is that many natural vegetable oils will help bring down cholesterol levels.

There is some controversy about how much fat to have in the diet. The American Heart Association recommends that fat should not exceed 10 percent of the total caloric intake. The National Research Council doesn't agree that that kind of restriction is necessary for the general population. If you read the actual research behind the cholesterol scare, you'll probably tend to agree with the National Research Council. You need fat in your diet. If you do not have high serum cholesterol, there is no reason to restrict cholesterol consumption. In fact, there is some evidence to indicate that low cholesterol levels may be associated with cancer and strokes.

Cholesterol is necessary to produce certain hormones. It is manufactured by the liver, so you will have cholesterol even if you do not eat it. This is why some people eat like rabbits and their cholesterol is still out in the stratosphere.

Refined and processed foods contribute to the cholesterol problem. Many packaged foods employ the use of hydrogenated oils. Hydrogenation increases the shelf life of the oil at the expense of turning it into a substance the body can't use, which screws up the fat metabolism. People using margarine to avoid cholesterol are doing themselves more harm than good. Margarine is just hydrogenated vegetable oil. A lot of prepackaged foods use these hydrogenated oils. Sometimes they have palm oil or coconut oil, which is highly saturated but is used because it is cheap.

Certain nutrients will bring down cholesterol levels, as will fiber and exercise. Many foods that contain cholesterol have nutrients that help the body put the cholesterol to good use. If you have a very high serum cholesterol or have a low HDL/LDL ratio, it may be necessary to limit your cholesterol intake.

Actually, there are things you can do that are more effective than just avoiding cholesterol. Many of the changes you make after reading this book will help, such as avoiding refined foods and hydrogenated oils, eating more fruits and vegetables, and exercising will probably do you more good than simply avoiding cholesterol.

Favorite Nutritional Disciplines

We select which foods we eat for many different reasons. The man I mentioned earlier avoided avocados because they were high in fat. What is really funny is that he had just finished telling me he didn't have a lot of time for lunch, so he usually grabbed something quick at a nearby hot dog stand (some of those low-fat hot dogs, no doubt).

What he does isn't so different from what many of us do. We learn little disciplines, such as staying away from butter, limiting egg consumption, not using salt, drinking diet pop (a horrible idea, but we'll talk about that one later), ordering the fried chicken sandwich instead of the burger (for what it's worth, breaded, deep-fat fried chicken has more fat than the burger), getting "cholesterol-free" French fries (honest — one of the fast food places now advertises this) or any number of other practices we've developed, only to let our cravings or low blood sugar lead us to ever worse dietary indiscretions.

One of the most common things a patient will say to me is, "I eat a pretty good diet. I stay away from red meat and eat a lot of chicken." Not that there's anything wrong with that. Chicken is a good source of protein. But there is a certain single-mindedness involved in this view. Often the person's "good diet" will consist of mostly meat and starch, probably a few diet colas throughout the week and very few vegetables. Their diet often lacks vitamins and minerals but, to their credit, it will be low in cholesterol and salt. As if there is something magic about staying away from cholesterol.

Too much cholesterol is not good, but people have become silly in their efforts to control it. The oat bran craze is a perfect example. Recently on the grocery shelf I saw a fried, saturated fat snack. On the label was a bright yellow banner, which overshadowed the name of the product. On the banner were the words "Contains Oat Bran." I assume they were marketing to someone fool enough to eat this saturated fat garbage and think it's healthy because it contains oat bran. Does oat bran magically wash cholesterol away? You could probably market horse manure, put a little oat bran in it and sell it as all natural and low fat food to help reduce cholesterol. Add a little aspartame (Nutra-Sweet) and you have a "diet food."

The media gets hold of an idea and it's sold to us as if it were the only issue on health and nutrition. This happens over and over again.

A long time ago the magic ingredient was iron. Recently calcium was a panacea. We were even sold an antacid as a calcium source, which is really ridiculous because you need acid to absorb calcium. We buy breakfast cereals that are loaded with sugar, chemicals and hydrogenated fat, just because they contain oat bran. We drink beverages and eat desserts that are strange mixtures of aspartame and other chemicals because they are low calorie. While we are loading up on chemicals and additives, we are avoiding eggs and other foods because they have cholesterol. Don't do this. Learn how your body works, apply your knowledge and eat whole foods. You won't have to worry about which multiple vitamin is giving you the most beta carotene to help you avoid colon cancer.

⊏⊐ *Remember there are no single issues in nutrition. There are no magic bullets. Cholesterol, salt, calcium, sugar and beta carotene are small parts of the whole picture. You do yourself a disservice if you pay an inordinate amount of attention to any one small aspect of nutrition.*

Learn How To Read Labels And Choose Your Food

Eat food. Sounds silly and obvious, doesn't it? Americans consume a lot of nonfoods and foods that have been altered to become, at best, non-nutritious and, at worst, poisonous. The ultimate nonfood is diet soda. It's a concoction of carbonated water, aspartame (NutraSweet) and coloring that has absolutely no food value.

There is another sugar-free, caffeine-free beverage that's available to you and it is considerabley cheaper: water. Drink water and not diet soda.

The Problem With Aspartame

Aspartame (NutraSweet) was put on the market in a hurry despite the objections of a federal panel that was concerned about the possibility of brain tumors. We're still waiting for the results of the human testing being done on this generation. It releases methanol (wood alcohol — which is poisonous) into the bloodstream. Aspartame can cause headaches, dizziness, blurred vision, nausea and a wide variety of other symptoms. If you must poison yourself and your children, at least choose familiar poisons, such as sugar. This way you won't be surprised by what happens.

I love the commercial that came out when aspartame was introduced. It said that it was made of "natural things," like part of a protein that was found in bananas and other good food. Actually, you could make the same claim for hydrogen cyanide. Hydrogen, nitrogen and carbon, the components of hydrogen cyanide, are found in bananas and other good things to eat.

Fats And Oils: Butter Versus Margarine

Margarine starts out as corn oil or some other vegetable oil, then the oil is hydrogenated so it becomes a solid at room temperature. Hydrogenation changes the oil's chemical configuration. The double bonds of the molecule are changed from a "cis" configuration to a "trans" configuration. The "trans" configuration is of no use to the body and is even toxic.

The difference between "cis" and "trans" molecular configurations is in the arrangement of the molecule. Chemically they contain the same things, but they are arranged differently. Chemically a potato and a two-by-four are the same, except for the way the molecules are arranged. Configuration is just as important in a fat molecule. Biomolecules are like fine machinery. How they are put together is as important as what is in them.

Margarine interferes with the body's ability to use essential fatty acids. Butter has taken a bad rap for its calories and cholesterol content. Butter is at least a food that the body can use, margarine is not. Few people realize that butter has the same number of calories as most margarines. (There are low-calorie margarines that have added water.) Butter may have cholesterol, but it also has lecithin and other nutrients that help the body metabolize cholesterol. Not that eating a lot of butter is good for you; it's just better than margarine.

Empty Calories Make You Overeat

Other nonfoods, such as cheese puffs and potato chips, have nothing to offer but fat, chemicals and empty calories. Set a potato chip on fire some time. Then ask yourself if you really want to eat something like that.

Consuming empty calories can cause us to overeat. One of the reasons we overeat is that there isn't enough food in our food. We become deficient in different vitamins, minerals and essential fatty acids. The body knows it needs something so it gets hungry, hoping that you have enough sense to eat something that has nutritional value. If you eat a meal of white bread, processed meat and a diet pop, the nutritional need still isn't met. If you attempt to satisfy hunger by eating empty calories, eating only to fill the stomach, you'll soon be hungry again. Not only that, but you'll feel lousy most of the time and gain weight.

The problem with junk food is not the extra calories. Eating junk food makes you want to eat more junk food. It is a cycle that is easier to break than you think. People who have spent some time eating healthfully find themselves now repulsed by junk food. It's just a matter of habit and making the effort to do without junk food until your tastes change.

Eat Like A Cave Man

When people come into my office for nutritional counseling, I tell them to go on a cave man diet. They come back complaining they can't find any brontosaurus steaks or mastodon chops. Then I have to explain that they shouldn't have any food that wasn't available to primitive man (or at least the early agrarian societies). If it comes in a bottle, box or can, stay away from it. It's not entirely practical advice to give to the busy urbanites who come into my office, but it is an ideal to strive for.

Eat food that is close to the state that nature provided. Your first choice is to eat whole grain right from the stalk. Your second choice is to eat it hand-milled at home. Your third choice is to eat it in bread or a cereal you make yourself. Your fourth choice is to eat whole grain bread made fresh with natural ingredients at a bakery you trust. Your fifth choice is to have it as a store-bought whole grain bread that may have a few additives in it. (Be careful to read the label when you buy whole wheat bread. Bread labeled as "wheat bread" is made with mostly white enriched flour with added food coloring to make it look brown.) Your sixth choice is to have the white enriched flour bread (stop before you get here). The next step is to have it pressed into a flake with a lot of added chemicals and sugar as a breakfast food. The next step is to add different chemicals and flavorings, deep fry it and have it as a snack food.

Foods in their natural state will satisfy your hunger more completely than processed foods. You will eat less of them and feel better. If you are used to convenience foods and eat a lot of packaged, processed and fast foods, changing to a more natural diet may be difficult for you, but not because the natural foods aren't enjoyable. It will be difficult because of time and having to learn how to eat all over again. Don't worry, just make small changes. Read your dietary diary and see where you can improve.

Little by little, start changing from processed foods to fresh and whole foods in their natural state. Buy whole grain bread instead of white. Instead of a frozen dinner, make your own casserole (this doesn't really take much more time than the frozen dinner).

Peanut butter was not available to the cave man, but it is not a bad food. It is best to grind fresh peanuts yourself. You can buy peanut butter in a jar, but buy a brand that is made only with peanuts. Smuckers makes one, so does Holsum. You can tell it has no added sugar or hydrogenated oil because the oil separates out. It's a little inconvenient, but it tastes better and is much better for you than the brands containing sugar and hydrogenated oil. Read the labels on the brands that don't have the oil separating out. You will find added sugar and hydrogenated oils. There is a peanut butter advertised by a former Mousketeer. I'm sure she's a nice lady, but don't take her nutritional advice when she says her brand has less sugar than leading brands. Apparently they don't consider Smuckers (which has no sugar) a leading brand.

How To Read A Product Label

Two places on any given package list what is in the product. The label, which has the information the manufacturer wants you to have, and the list of ingredients, which the government makes the manufacturer tell you. The ingredients are listed with the most plentiful first, second most plentiful ingredient listed second and so on.

On the ingredients list you learn that honey-labeled cereals have a lot of sugar but not a lot of honey. Breakfast cereals are great items to compare the marketing on their labels to their ingredients lists. Let's look at one that shall remain nameless. In small letters on the bottom it says "low in sodium." The graphics on the package look as if the cereal was made during the turn of the century — with old-fashioned goodness. The ingredients are listed in the following order: rolled oats, brown sugar, crisp rice, sunflower oil, dried dates, almond pieces, coconut, honey, sugar, sesame seeds, salt, applesauce, soy lecithin, crushed oranges, malt syrup, cinnamon and vanilla extract.

Lots of good stuff, right? You'll notice the second ingredient is brown sugar. Everyone seems to think that brown sugar is healthier than white sugar; it's not. Brown sugar is just caramelized, or heated, white sugar. This product has sugar as its second most plentiful ingredient. Sugar and malt syrup are also listed elsewhere. So, in total, sugar is listed three times, in three different forms on the label. I'm not saying they're doing it here, but this is one way manufacturers can have a product with sugar as its most plentiful ingredient without having to list sugar first.

You'll see this in a lot of products. The label will read: sugar, dextrose, maltose, brown sugar. All of these things are sugar. Malt syrup is sugar. By breaking it up like that, the manufacturer can keep from listing sugar first or second on the ingredient label. Usually if the word ends in "ose" it's a sugar. Dextrose, maltose, lactose, sucrose, glucose and fructose are all sugars.

Let's try another label. We have a popular salad dressing that advertises itself as being good for your heart. The label indicates the dressing is 91 percent fat free and cholesterol free. Sounds like just the thing for someone trying to take care of his or her health. The ingredients are listed as follows: water, partially hydrogenated soybean oil, cultured nonfat buttermilk solids, sugar, modified food starch, salt, natural flavors, sodium caseinate, vinegar, phosphoric acid, onion (dehydrated), garlic (dehydrated), monosodium glutamate (enhances flavor [actually tricks your nervous system into thinking that it tastes good]), propylene glycol alginate, mono and diglycerides, sorbic acid, lactic acid, spice, artificial flavor, xanthan gum, disodium inositate and disodium guanylate, parsley (dehydrated), calcium disodium EDTA, THBQ and citric acid.

Just what are you eating here? I'll give you a little synopsis. The information has been obtained from David Steinman's *Diet for a Poisoned Planet* and Ruth Winter's *Consumer's Dictionary of Food Additives*.

Water: The most plentiful ingredient in this product. What's an easy way to make something that's 20 percent fat into something that's 10 percent fat? Add 50 percent water, it's low-fat and it's cheap (and so far, it's reasonably safe, but we won't be able to take that for granted for very long).

Unfortunately, you don't know how much fat would have been in the dressing if the water wasn't added. Manufacturers are not required to tell the amounts of the ingredients in their products. They are merely required to list them with the most plentiful ingredient first, second most plentiful second, and so forth.

Partially hydrogenated soybean oil: Better than completely hydrogenated, right? Wrong! Hydrogenation turns an unsaturated fat into a saturated one. It also turns it into something the body can't really use. (Udo Erasmus' book, *Fats and Oils* is a good source for information about hydrogenation.)

Cultured nonfat buttermilk solids: Probably better than illiterate nonfat buttermilk solids. Actually, it's much like powdered milk.

Sugar: Replaces some of the taste lost from watering it down.

Modified food starch: This is starch that has been chemically altered to make it water soluble. Several different chemicals are used, propylene oxide, succinic anhydride, 1-octenyl succinic anhydride, aluminum sulfate and sodium hydroxide. You have no way of knowing what was used. In Steinman's book, he was most concerned about the aluminum sulfate because of the possible link between aluminum and Alzheimer's disease.

Natural flavors: According to Ruth Winter's *Consumer's Dictionary of Food Additives,* the FTC considers something natural if only minimal processing, such as peeling, homogenizing, baking and things that can be done in the kitchen, has been done to the food. Also the food cannot have anything synthetic or any added chemicals. Beyond that, you don't know what these natural flavors are.

Sodium caseinate: This is the principal protein of cow's milk.

Vinegar: Finally something you can recognize as a food that you would find in your own kitchen.

Phosphoric acid: This is an acid made from phosphate rock. The FDA considers it safe. Steinman makes the point that you can clean rust off a chrome bumper with it.

Salt: Something else that is familiar.

Onion and garlic (dehydrated): More food. This could get to be a habit.

Monosodium glutamate: Causes "Chinese Restaurant Syndrome" (chest pain, numbness and headache after eating). Causes brain damage in young rodents. Female animals treated with MSG had fewer pregnancies and smaller litters.

Propylene glycol alginate: Derived from seaweed. The FDA considers it safe.

Mono and diglycerides: According to Steinman, these can occur in nature, but are usually synthetically made. In his book, Steinman cites studies that show certain types of mono and diglycerides have caused decreased growth in mice, others have caused enlarged kidneys and decrease in the size of testes. (The poor mice probably are not sure whether they're coming or going.)

Sorbic acid: This is acetic acid. It is relatively harmless.

Lactic acid: This occurs naturally in sour milk. This is regarded as safe by the FDA.

Spice: It now has sugar and spice (and everything nice?).

Artificial Flavor: By definition, something not found in nature, although it may have components that are found in nature. Whatever it is, the manufacturer has opted not to tell you in detail what the substance is; sort of a mystery chemical.

Xanthan gum: Produced by fermentation of corn sugar. Thickens and helps it pour well. No known toxicity.

Disodium inositate: A flavor enhancer. No known toxicity.

Parsley (dehydrated): Another food.

Calcium disodium EDTA: Ethylenediaminetetraacetate (no kidding, I know it looks like my daughter played with the computer keys for the last few minutes, but that's really the name of this stuff). Steinman says that it is used to bind to materials that are undesirable in food. It hides metallic tastes and other undesirable flavors and colors in the food. This means that the dressing might taste a little weird (small wonder) without the EDTA. Steinman also expresses concern that this can bind to minerals and rob your body of them.

THBQ: Tertiary butylhydroquinone, food manufacturers had a hard time getting the FDA to approve this. According to Ruth Winter's book, death has occurred from ingestion of five grams. Eating one gram can cause nausea, vomiting, ringing in the ears, delirium, a sense of suffocation and collapse.

Citric acid: One of the safer additives according to Steinman.

Aren't you glad that you're avoiding all that nasty vegetable oil by buying this stuff? This is an important lesson for you to learn because a lot of "food" sold to people trying to lose weight has a lot of chemicals. Actually the word "lite" is an ancient Sanskrit word menaing: "full of chemicals."

This dressing has less oil, as promised by the label. But it does have a lot of chemicals and a fair amount of sugar. It has partially hydrogenated oil. Compare it to a more "fattening" dressing found refrigerated in your store's produce department, Marie's Ranch Dressing. The ingredients are: soybean oil, fresh buttermilk, whole eggs, egg yolks, distilled vinegar, sugar, salt, spices (dehydrated), garlic (dehydrated), onion (dehydrated), xanthan gum (a natural food fiber). I'm sure that this is no bargain in the realm of calories, and it does contain some sugar, but you're better off with Marie's than you are with the first dressing (you can water it down yourself.)

Food Additives And
Why You Should Avoid Them

The average American gets ten pounds of additives per year. We don't yet fully understand the health implications of this. The only studies ever done are on single additives. To my knowledge, no one has studied the cumulative effect of all of these chemicals. Until the effects are known, you're better off with the nonchemical version.

There's a poster available from the Center for Science in the Public Interest that rates the food additives. The poster lists which additives are "safe" and which are dangerous. I have a degree in chemistry and I have the poster. My criteria are: If I can't pronounce it, if it has too many syllables or if it is listed just by its initials (MSG, EDTA, BHT, etc.), I don't want to eat it. Actually, I'm just lazy. Some of these things are relatively benign, but if you are going to eat packaged foods, please learn what they contain. If you can motivate yourself to eat whole fresh foods, you won't have to worry about labeling. Ruth Winter's book, *A Consumer's Dictionary of Food Additives*, contains a very complete list of additives.

Substances added to food that are usually not a problem are things like riboflavin, thiamine, niacin, ascorbic acid, alpha tocopherol, lecithin and beta carotene. These are nutrients. Adding them to food usually does no harm. The vitamins are not as good as those provided by nature, but they shouldn't hurt you.

Citric acid, sodium citrate, sorbic (acetic) acid, lactic acid and fumaric acid are also fine. They are lightweight organic acids often found in nature. Alginates, ghatti, gum tragacanth, karaya, locust bean, fucelleran and carob are plant products and relatively benign. Casein is a protein and is harmless to most people. Calcium proprionate, sodium proprionate and sodium benzoate are preservatives that have been around a while and have established a fairly safe track record.

There may be other relatively harmless additives, but by no stretch of the imagination am I saying that some additives are good. You are still better off with food in its natural state, but this is the real world and most of us are not that disciplined. So if you eat packaged foods, make it a point to know what is in the package.

As a general rule, I stay away from any artificial colorings (often they are listed on a package as a color followed by a number, such as blue #2 or red #40). These things are always being pronounced "safe" only to be taken of the market later. (Remember the red M&Ms?)

Usually you want to avoid chemicals described by three or more letters such a BVO (brominated vegetable oil — avoid this one like the plague), BHT (butylated hydroxytoulene), BHA (butylated hydroxyanhiosole), THBQ (tertiary butylhydroquinone) and MSG (monosodium glutamate). It is as if organic chemists are somehow stuck in the Roosevelt era; they love those three-letter names. BVO, BHE, BHT and THBQ you especially want to avoid. MSG is a flavoring that works by triggering a response in your nervous system. It can make you dizzy and nauseous and can also give you heart palpitations and perhaps even headaches and hives. MSG is also found in "hydrolyzed vegetable protein." Everyone reacts badly to MSG. Some are more tolerant so it takes a lot more of it to make them sick. Others, who are more sensitive to the flavoring suffer from "Chinese Restaurant Syndrome" when they consume small amounts. I don't know about you, but I really resent having neuroactive chemicals put into my food so that it will be lip-smacking good.

Stay away from foods with "artificial flavor." It's a vague term. Usually when you see those words, they're in a food you should avoid for other reasons.

Avoid nitrites that are found in ham, bologna, salami and other processed luncheon meats. These are chemical-

and fat-intensive foods that you want to steer clear of. Turkey ham, turkey salami and turkey bologna may have less fat, but they are still loaded with nitrites.

Sulfites (sulfur dioxide, sodium bisulfate and sodium metabisulfate) should be avoided, especially by asthmatics. Sulfites are often found in dried fruits, especially apricots.

Food Additives And Allergies

From a strict weight-loss point of view, chemicals don't add a lot of calories to your food. But from the standpoint of staying healthy, it makes a lot of sense to stay away from them. One possible cause of the epidemic increase in allergies is the increase of chemicals in our food. Even those listed here as benign may be implicated in allergic reactions and some even contribute to hyperactivity in children. It may seem as if we are straying from the topic of weight loss here but not really. You will feel better if you limit your chemical consumption. You will be less likely to overeat if you eat only whole and natural foods.

A number of health problems have arisen due to the overprocessing of foods. One of them is obesity. Essential fatty acids, some of the most important nutrients, are not found in sufficient amounts in modern diets. A lack of essential fatty acids can cause you to crave fried and other high-fat foods. We do get a fair amount of arachadonic acid (an essential fatty acid found in meats and dairy food), but linoleic acid is often missing from our diets. In fact, lacking linoleic acid will often cause you to crave dairy or meat products but they won't satisfy a need for linoleic acid.

Cholesterol And The "Right" Oils And Fats

Because of processing methods, most of the oils and fats in our diets are, at best, empty calories and, at worst, toxic. Natural oils are very easily destroyed by light and heat. Most of the oils used in cooking, those lightweight oils seen in clear bottles on your grocer's shelf, are not good for you. The oil is extracted from the vegetable using either heat or chemicals that destroy the essential fatty acid content. Adjectives such as "polyunsaturated," "cholesterol-free" and "pure corn oil" are meaningless. What really matters is how the oil was produced. It should be "cold pressed," but even that is not enough. Some of these oils are heated after they are extracted. The oil should never reach a temperature of more than 50° centigrade during its manufacture. It should be stored in a dark container. Refrigerate it when you get it home. Squeezing the contents of a vitamin E capsule into the oil will help preserve it.

It's funny how everyone is paranoid about cholesterol, but they consume hydrogenated and commercially processed oils without a second thought.

Are We As Healthy As Our Grandparents?

At the turn of the century one American in 30 died of cancer. Today it is one in five. In 1900 cardiovascular disease was responsible for one death in seven, today 50 percent of the population dies from it. Experts wring their hands and blame animal fats and cholesterol. While it is true that cholesterol consumption had been increasing in the first half of this century, it hasn't increased enough to account for the increase in heart disease. Cholesterol consumption has decreased steadily in the last 20 years without significantly changing these statistics. To place the sole blame on cholesterol for the increase in heart disease is silly.

What has increased since 1900 is the hydrogenation of oils, processing of foods and the addition of chemicals in our food and our environment. At the turn of the century, salad and cooking oil were extracted from flax seed and the process involved no heat. People had an abundance of essential fatty acids in their diets. Today we consume fewer calories and about the same amount of animal fat as at the turn of the century, but we are more obese, and we are dropping like flies from cancer and heart disease.

Getting Back To Basics

Weaning yourself from packaged and processed foods will be difficult. We are all so busy and there is so much to learn (with the learning made difficult by the fact that no one agrees on nutritional issues).

Getting quality food takes time and effort in today's fast-food society. Start by making small changes. Choose turkey breast instead of nitrite-loaded salami. Select whole wheat bread instead of white. Eat oatmeal instead of a sugar-loaded cereal. Little by little learn what is in the food you eat and always strive to make better food decisions.

Removing the added sugars and hydrogenated oils will help you lose weight. Limiting the chemicals will help your general health. If you have headaches, PMS, fatigue, digestive problems or allergies, this is a section you should pay particular attention to. Losing weight is difficult if you don't feel well.

What Food Labels Don't Tell You

My wife and I have been working hard at getting the additives out of the food we eat, but it's not easy. Occasionally we get fooled by a label. We've been buying a whole grain cereal with almonds and raisins because the box says no added sugar, which is wonderful. (Go to your grocery store and try to find a boxed cereal without added sugar.) It tastes great, so we've been buying it every week. But it seemed to taste sweet for a sugar-free cereal. Our mistake was to assume that "no added sugar" meant "sugar-free." Although the claim is no added sugar, the cereal does have malt flavoring added, which contains sugar. This company's wheat flakes have about two grams of sugar per ounce, which is about six and a half percent. That's not as much as most of the others but it certainly isn't sugar free.

My wife and I have a one-year-old daughter who drinks a lot of juice instead of sugared drinks. Trying to make it easy on ourselves and not haul two gallons of juice from the store one week, we bought a white grape juice concentrate. I was taken by surprise here. I always thought juice was juice. If it had sugar added, it becomes juice cocktail, juice drink or fruit drink. I was wrong. In very small letters above the words "white grape juice" was the word "sweetened."

Manufacturers are not proud of having sugar in their products, so you'll never see a big yellow banner on the label saying, "LOADED WITH SUGAR!" They tend to go to great lengths to hide it. If you don't read carefully, you'll consume more sugar than you intend to. I almost bought a grape concentrate because in big letters it said, "ALL NATURAL," but in tiny letters it said, "juice cocktail," which meant it has sugar. Apparently sugar is a natural ingredient. There is a "sugar-free" version but it has aspartame, which is worse.

One popular brand did trick me with its labeling. I wanted to get my daughter some white grape juice, not wanting to give her purple grape juice (no health reason here, a purple liquid is something you do not want to give to a one-year-old). I bought "100 percent White Grape Juice" (with vitamin C). No sugar added, written right there on the label. Sounds good. I got it home and read the ingredients. It has potassium metabisulfite added (a sulfite). If it is 100 percent juice and it has this chemical in it, that must mean there is more than 100 percent of stuff in this bottle. I've had one or two math classes and they left me with the impression that this wasn't possible. Silly me, I thought that 100 percent juice meant that there was nothing but juice in the bottle.

This product has sulfite added to it. If my child were asthmatic, this could have sent her to the hospital. People have died from sulfites added to food. So read the ingredients; even "trusted" brand names can't be trusted.

I'm not trying to get you to become some sort of fanatic. I know many people who are much stricter about their diets than I am. You will find some kind of middle ground with which you are comfortable. Don't feel pressured by what is in this section, and don't feel that you have to go off the deep end and start eating things with little or no taste. Just gradually make healthy decisions.

Eat Lots Of Fresh Fruit And Vegetables

Fruit and vegetables make great snacks. They will satisfy your hunger pangs without adding a lot of calories to your diet. You should have seven servings per day. That's four cups of vegetables and three servings of fruit per day (more if you want it). Fruit and vegetables are high in bulk and fiber and will make you feel full, so you'll have less of an appetite for fattening foods. The fiber will also reduce the fat and calories you absorb from other foods. Eating a lot of fruit and vegetables will improve your digestion, speed up your bowel transit time and decrease the toxicity in your colon. Your health and energy will increase and your chances of developing bowel cancer will decrease.

Fruits and vegetables are high in vitamins and minerals and low in calories. You'd have to eat seven cups of raw spinach to get the same number of calories as that in a Mars bar. But that would still be no comparison. Because of all of the fiber in spinach, you'd never absorb that many calories. And spinach has beta carotene, the latest buzz word in the fight against cancer.

The vitamins and minerals found in fresh fruits and vegetables will help you reach your weight goal. Much overeating is an attempt by the body to supply nutrients that are missing from the food. If you are eating a refined, vitamin-deficient diet, you will overeat. If you eat plenty of fresh fruit and vegetables, your tendency to overeat will lessen.

Two-thirds of a cup of raw broccoli has only 32 calories and contains 113 milligrams of vitamin C, 2,500 international units of vitamin A, plus calcium, phosphorus, potassium and magnesium. George Bush doesn't like broccoli. It probably tastes bitter to him. A kinder and gentler cook would peel the stalks before cooking them in a little bit of lemon. That would make it taste much better. Mr. Bush would be so estatic, he'd see a thousand points of light shining above the dinner table. (Tastes good with a little quail, too).

I tell my patients to eat four cups of vegetables and they come back and tell me that they don't have time to eat a lot of junk food because they're so busy trying to get all those vegetables down. You won't miss what you think you love to eat if you're well fed all of the time.

⊏⊐ *Eat all you want. Keep fresh celery, carrots, radishes, apples, pears, peaches, kiwi fruit, okra, passion fruit, kumquats or whatever you like on hand. Make sure there is plenty at home and at work. Snack and don't let yourself get too hungry. You make your worst dietary decisions when you're hungry. Eating will also help speed up your metabolism if you are one of those people who look at food and get fat. If you are a nervous eater, snacking on fresh fruits and vegetables will keep your mouth busy, without adding a lot of extra calories.*

Absolutely Avoid Commercially Fried Foods

This is a health tip as well as a weight-loss tip. There are so many reasons not to eat fried food that it's hard to know where to begin. There are a lot of extra calories in fried foods, probably a lot more than you realize. There are roughly three times the calories in French fries as there are in boiled potatoes. There are 76 calories in a medium-sized boiled potato (100 grams). A 100-gram serving of French fries has about 206 calories. A broiled chicken breast has about 288 calories. The same weight of fried, boneless chicken has 457 calories. That's 169 needless calories, almost 60 percent more calories than the plain chicken. The grease and starch in the fried breading have absolutely no food value. It isn't necessary to starve yourself to lose weight, just give up the needless extra calories.

Deep fat friers are hot all day long. Some places don't even change their oil every day. The heat breaks down the oil and creates a wide variety of carcinogens and other toxic substances. Even ignoring the possibility of increasing your chances for cancer and heart disease, these fats are a terrible burden on your liver and gall bladder.

Eating fried foods causes you to crave more of the same. Calories are the least of your worries when it comes to eating fried foods.

Buy Organically Grown
Foods Whenever Possible

American agriculture consists of dumping chemical fertilizer on overused, depleted soil, spreading poison on it to keep insects from eating the crops and, in many cases, irradiating produce to keep it "fresh." Personally I'm suspicious of anything that bugs avoid, no matter how safe the government and food industry tell me it is.

Bigger obscenities are committed on meats and poultry. Animals are fed steroids and antibiotics. Chickens are fed hormones and not allowed to move about freely. They are literally turned into egg-laying factories. Disease is common, so they are given antibiotics (sold in a feed store, given at the discretion of the farmer). The government inspector spends an average of only two seconds per chicken.

If you've ever eaten a chicken that has been allowed to roam freely and not fed any drugs, it's like eating a different kind of food from a supermarket chicken. The eggs from these chickens have very hard shells. The yolks are amber because they are so rich in vitamin A, and the yolks are hard to break. You won't find yourself having scrambled eggs when you really wanted over-easy, just because you broke the yolk. These eggs taste amazingly better and they even have less cholesterol. Comparing the pale, weak-shelled eggs found in the supermarket to the eggs of range chickens is like comparing styrofoam to cheese. Don't be fooled by brown eggs — just because the shell is brown doesn't mean that the egg came from a range chicken. Try buying "nest eggs" in your supermarket. If you can buy eggs directly from a farmer, that's even better.

The difference between organic meats and vegetables and their supermarket counterparts is also very marked. These foods are harder to find and sometimes more expensive, but they are not expensive compared to processed and packaged food. If you were to figure out a ratio between cost and food value, the organic foods would be cheaper.

Dairy producers are trying to get permission to feed cattle Bovine Growth Hormone without having to tell consumers that the milk came from a cow that was fed this chemical. The proponents of food irradiation would prefer that the consumers not know if food is irradiated. Food irradiation is basically exposing food to radioactive waste.

The folks who bring you MSG are very upset that a bill in Maine was passed requiring restaurants to inform the public when MSG is added to a dish. All this is happening because those who want to feed hormones to cows, irradiate food and give us "Chinese Restaurant Syndrome" are afraid that if consumers know what has been done to their food, sales will go down. There are people spending money and using political influence to keep you from knowing what is in your food. Remember to follow these events closely when they happen in your area. Support CSPI. They are very active in fighting for your right to know what is in your food.

Back to losing weight . . . remember losing weight? Eating organic food will enable you to enjoy plain foods without relying on butter, sauces, dressings and cheese for flavor. Organic meats and produce are richer in vitamins and minerals and therefore will satisfy your hunger more readily than foods not organically produced.

▭ *Also, we are back to the topic of chemicals in the food. You cannot completely avoid chemicals, but you should minimize them. Food allergies and digestive problems may be caused by them. If you don't feel good, are fatigued, have allergies, Epstein-Barr virus or any chronic health problems, taking the toxic burden of chemicals off your liver becomes important in your quest for thinness. It's hard to concentrate on losing weight if you don't feel well.*

Learn To Control Cravings

Fried Foods

One very common craving is fried foods. This was one of mine. Very often you crave fried foods because you need essential fatty acids or are deficient in an oil-soluble vitamin. For some reason your body doesn't seem to know the difference between saturated fat, grease and essential fatty acids. Oil, grease . . . it's all the same to your body (until it tries to put the substance to use).

The reason for this is that you're the owner of the same body as a cave man or woman. There weren't artificially hydrogenated oils and deep fat frying in prehistoric times. Anything in the cave man's diet that was oily contained essential fatty acids. When he was deficient in oils, he developed a taste for oily foods. You do the same thing, except you eat hydrogenated oils and fried foods. So you crave fried foods and things with hydrogenated oils in them, which actually make the situation worse.

There are other symptoms that accompany a lack of essential fatty acids, such as muscle soreness or weakness, dry skin or eczema, itchy skin, dandruff, acne or even allergies.

If any of these symptoms are a problem for you or if you crave fried or greasy foods, you should eat foods high in essential fatty acids such as avocados, legumes and nuts. (Buy them in the shell and raw, not roasted.) You absolutely should avoid products that contain hydrogenated vegetable oil, especially margarine and mayonnaise, and fried foods. These make the problem worse by interfering with your body's ability to metabolize essential oils. Read labels.

In my practice I often use essential fatty acid supplements, such as omega-3 and omega-6. It's hard to get into explaining them without turning this into a biochemistry lesson. I use black currant seed oil or flax seed supplement with B6. Generally the patient takes about 500 milligrams of the oil three times per day. It works; the cravings stop.

Other foods you may crave if you are deficient in fatty acids are dairy products, especially butter and cheese, greasy meats like sausages and hamburgers or mayonnaise. Sometimes craving dairy products indicates an allergy.

Sugar And Chocolate

Another food people often crave is sugar. Very often these people are hypoglycemic. The blood sugar drops and their bodies know that a can of cola will pick it back up. If you use the sugar to raise your blood sugar, you'll just want more sugar later. Eating fruit or other healthy snacks every two hours will eliminate this craving. You will be amazed how easily.

Chocolate cravings can be fat or sugar cravings. Chocolate bars are made with hydrogenated oil, so they may be craved by a person who needs fatty acids. They have a lot of sugar, so they are craved by the hypoglycemic. Chocolate is also a common allergen.

Nutritional Deficiencies And Overeating

Sometimes needing certain nutrients will create cravings or the desire to overeat. People who need support for their adrenal glands will often crave salt. Those who need trace minerals will often bite their nails. Other nutritional deficiencies may cause a person to overeat. It's as if the body wants to keep eating until it finally gets what it needs. Eating plenty of organic fruits and green vegetables will help supply the body with enough vitamins and minerals to make this less of a problem. Vitamin supplements may also help.

⊏▭▭⊐ *Not digesting food well may cause you to overeat and crave all kinds of food. Eating food that you do not digest well is like having "the check in the mail." Even though the stomach is full, the body's needs are still not satisfied. You are still hungry. Digestive enzymes, hydrochloric acid or other supplements may be needed. Sometimes the foods that are hard to digest may be identified and avoided.*

D

Limiting Caloric Intake The Right Way

We've been talking about calories throughout the book. It is not necessary to restrict your caloric intake severely in order to lose weight, but it does help to be aware of calories and to avoid the unnecessary ones. In the last section you've seen how you can eliminate extra calories by avoiding fried food and sugar, although the worst thing about these foods is not the extra calories. The problem is that they make you crave more junk food. (Like the ad says, "Bet ya can't eat just one.") If you overeat or you are a nervous eater, the information in this section will help you.

The calorie is a unit of energy. In chemistry a calorie is the amount of heat required to raise the temperature of one gram (milliliter) of water one degree centigrade. When the term is used in dieting, what is called a calorie is actually a kilocalorie. A kilocalorie is the amount of heat needed to raise the temperature of one liter of water one degree centigrade. One pound of fat has approximately 3,500 calories (kilocalories) of energy and is roughly the amount of energy it would take to bring nine gallons of water from ice to steam.

Fifty pounds of fat is enough energy for a 180-pound person to walk from Flagstaff, Arizona, to Gary, Indiana (although God knows why he would want to do that). If you're in a hurry to lose the 50 pounds, this will take you about 450 hours. That's not counting calories gained from resting and meals. Figuring that in, you'll probably end up in Minsk.

The first and most commonly used method of weight loss is calorie reduction. By now you know how futile that is. You don't fail to lose weight because you can't stay on a 1,200-calorie diet. You fail to lose weight because of all of the extra calories you consume when you are not dieting. *You will lose weight if you eat only when you are hungry, if you exercise regularly and if you avoid eating empty calories.*

Eating 2,400 calories per day is right around average (depending on your weight and sex). Think of those calories as money to spend on nutrients. Make sure you get your money's worth.

If you spend 230 calories to have a chocolate bar, it's a lot like spending $230 on a broken record player that only plays at 78 RPM. Having flank steak, a potato and green beans would be like buying a CD player.

Some of us consume calories we don't really want or need by eating nervously, eating more than we really need to fill ourselves up at a meal and by eating too fast.

If you keep track of your caloric intake during your program, you may notice that you're automatically eating fewer calories than before, especially if you've increased your consumption of fresh fruits and vegetables. Fruits and vegetables are high-bulk, low-calorie foods that will fill you up and keep you from eating more fattening foods. If you ate 230 calories in the form of fresh spinach, you would have to eat almost two pounds. That would be the equivalent of getting the whole stereo system, with the CD player and a pair of ear-splitting speakers for $230.

The average American eats between 2,200 and 2,500 calories per day. You don't have to reduce that amount to 1,200 or 1,500 calories to lose weight. In fact, if you are eating too few calories, your metabolism may already be too slow and you'll just make your situation worse by further limiting food intake.

If you consume too many calories — in the 3,000 or 4,000 calorie per day range — some of the suggestions in this section will help you. If you overeat, and you feel that you have no control over your appetite, it is very important that you control the quality of what you eat by following what is in the previous section. If self-control is still too difficult for you at this point, it is possible that you have allergies or digestive problems, but we will cover those topics later.

Eat Slowly.
Chew Your Food Thoroughly

Chew your food thoroughly until it is liquid. Put your fork down between mouthfuls. That will keep you from using your fork like a shovel and swallowing large chunks of food whole. Stop eating at several points during the meal, just for a minute or so.

Conversation at dinner is nice. Conversing causes you to eat slowly and to stop eating for brief periods of time (unless you're eating with someone who won't let you get in a word edgewise).

Eating slowly accomplishes a few things that will help you in your quest for a thin healthy body.

- You will digest your food better if you chew it well.
- Your saliva has amylase, which breaks down carbohydrates.
- You will increase your blood sugar at a slow, steady rate, which will allow you to feel full sooner.

Chewing is the first phase of digestion and doing a thorough job of it will make things easy for the pancreas and other digestive organs. It's easy for your enzymes to break down food that isn't swallowed in big chunks. If you're eating lots of fresh raw vegetables, your digestion will get some enzymatic assistance from them. If you tend to have gas and to bloat after meals, thoroughly chewing your food is very important.

People who skip meals become too hungry and, as a result, inhale their food. They then end up eating more than they would if they ate regularly during the day.

Another benefit of eating slowly is that plain foods taste better to you than they do when you inhale your food. A lot of the fat and calories we consume comes from dressing up our food. Heavy salad dressings, cream sauces and butter add a lot of calories and fat to our meals. If you take your time while eating, the subtle flavor of plain, fresh vegetables is very enjoyable.

⊏══⊐ *If you eat slowly, you will become full much sooner than you would if you inhale your food. If you eat too fast you will continue to eat after you're full because your body's mechanism to recognize that it is full doesn't work fast enough. This causes you to overeat.*

Learn To Like Plain Foods

If you automatically think of broccoli as good only if it is smothered in cheese sauce or if you only enjoy vegetables when they are overcooked and dripping with butter, eating slowly will help you to appreciate the taste of the pure vegetable.

Lemon and other low-calorie seasonings will enhance the flavor of vegetables without smothering them. We consume a lot of unnecessary calories and fat in dressings and sauces. Brown gravy has about 164 calories in a quarter cup. Hollandaise has 180 calories in a quarter cup, with 18 grams of fat. Creamy French dressing has about 70 calories in a tablespoon. This is not to say that you should never have salad dressing or gravy, but you should cut down on the amount you now consume. Make it a habit to have dressings and sauces served to you on the side and remember to use them sparingly. If you can do without them, so much the better — but don't force yourself.

Many of us don't appreciate the taste of plain vegetables. I see a lot of diet intake sheets in my office and very few people eat enough dark green vegetables. Many eat salads consisting mainly of iceberg lettuce. There's nothing really wrong with iceberg lettuce, but it doesn't have the food value of spinach or Romaine. In fact, it has very little food value at all.

Eating slowly will help you to enjoy the taste of many plain foods. There are subtle flavors that can only be enjoyed when the food is eaten slowly. Choosing organically grown foods will also make you appreciate plain foods.

Our disdain for vegetables and our desire to smother their flavors isn't entirely our fault. A lot of it has to do with the quality of produce available to us.

We have a friend from Greece who finds that food in Greece tastes better than the food in the United States. This attitude is perceived by her American friends as the "Everything is better in Greece" attitude. (I have a lot of patients who agree with her, but they put it, "Everything is better in grease.") My friend used to say that the produce here tasted like wood and that food was better in Greece. We teased her about it and told her that she was just homesick. Then we went to Greece with her and her husband. She was right, the food did taste better. It was as if everything came fresh from your own garden.

A lot of the produce in the United States is fairly tasteless. Who hasn't bought a nice big red perfect-looking apple only to bite into it and have it taste like sawdust? I bought some large cantaloupes the other day. Inside they were the color of a manila folder, hard as wood, dry and tasteless.

Agriculture is big business in this country. We produce a lot of food. When the soil becomes depleted, chemical fertilizers are used. Adding nitrogen to the soil isn't really harmful to the food, but a lot of the things a plant needs to grow are not added; instead, chemical fertilizers are used. So you end up with big, pretty-looking, tasteless food, with fewer vitamins and minerals than its organically grown counterpart. It's no wonder we like our produce smothered in cheese, salad dressings and sauces.

You can shop around and find better produce. Go to farm stands or places that sell organic produce. If you have time, grow it yourself. (You'll even get a little extra exercise.)

With some effort you will enjoy plain vegetables much more. After a while you become good at selecting produce. You won't need to smother your vegetables in cheese or ranch dressing, and you will be consuming more healthy vitamins and minerals. You will also find that eating foods rich in vitamins and minerals will help you to control food cravings.

Don't Clean Your Plate

The ancient Celtics (before Larry Bird) used to leave their last morsel of food or drink for the wood nymphs. So don't finish all of your food. You'll not only please the wood nymphs, but you'll also break the habit of eating when you're already full simply to avoid wasting food.

My parents were newlyweds during the Depression. My father was out of work for over a year. They got their start in life being very poor. As a result, in our house you simply did not throw food away. To this day, even if someone gives me an obscenely large portion, I'll finish it.

At home I have solved this problem with Tupperware. It's the greatest invention to find its way into the modern kitchen. Tupperware enables me to store the food in the refrigerator until it becomes moldy so I don't feel guilty throwing it away.

Storing food in Tupperware does lead to a waiting contest between my wife and me. Our Tupperware is opaque, and after a few days you forget what's in it. After a few more days, you're afraid to open it. It then sits in the back of the refrigerator until one of us gets brave enough to open it or we run out of clean Tupperware. Opening one of these containers can be quite an adventure. One time something jumped out of the container, killed our dog and escaped into an air vent. We don't know what it was, but we're waiting for Sigourney Weaver to come and kill it.

Cleaning your plate to avoid wasting food will frequently cause you to overeat. Since you're eating when you're hungry and not denying yourself food, you have to make the effort not to consume food when you're not hungry. Forcing food down when you're already full is just another way to get extra calories. Purposely leaving a small amount of food will help you to break this habit. If waste is an issue, take smaller portions and use Tupperware.

Don't Clean Someone Else's Plate

This is repetitive, I know, but it's for my mother-in-law. She's not obese by any stretch of the definition of the word. But like most of us, she'd be happier if she weighed a little less. She used to be extremely thin, like my wife. She gained her weight after she had children, not from the actual pregnancies, but from finishing the food that the kids didn't eat.

Don't Eat If You're Not Hungry

Seems pretty obvious, doesn't it? A lot of us are nervous eaters and consume food that we don't realize we're eating. If you keep a regular food diary, you'll notice how this adds up. Sampling food while cooking, eating in front of the TV, overeating at parties and on holidays and other such habits need to be broken.

Some people tend to eat a lot when they're under stress. Find some other way to deal with stress. (No, don't start smoking.) I tend to eat when I'm under stress and to unconsciously nibble when I'm not really hungry. When I write or study and I get excited about what I'm doing, I tend to want to eat. I solved this problem for myself by buying toys. I'm now pretty good with a yo-yo (probably makes me a yo-yo dieter) and I've learned how to juggle (my daughter loves it). In my office I have a dart board on the wall in the back and a miniature basketball hoop over the wastebasket.

Granted doing rock the cradle with a yo-yo and throwing darts are not for everyone, but the idea is to find a substitute for nervous eating. Gum works for some people.

⊏⊐ *This is an area where visualizing will help. Just picture your ideal self finding other things to do besides eating. If you catch yourself absentmindedly eating, take a minute to remind yourself what you're working for. If you absolutely cannot stop nibbling, limit yourself to carrot and celery sticks or plain popcorn.*

Beware Of Triggers

I'm not blaming Roy Rogers' late horse for your spare tire. A trigger is something that makes you eat inappropriately. A bad day at work, a football game, a fight with your spouse or a trip to the movies can all be triggers. For some people, waking up is a trigger. My favorite trigger used to be the TV set. I'd have my wife bring me the phone. (Once I'd settled into the little canyon I created at my end of the couch, it was a major effort to get it myself.) Then I'd call for pizza. Deep-dish, Chicago-style pizza with enough cheese to spackle your arteries shut and a variety of greasy meats to give it an interesting consistency, a veritable cholesterol orgy. We'd eat until we were stuffed and leave the leftover pizza on the coffee table. In a half hour we'd eat some more.

Your daily diet diary will help you to identify inappropriate eating. Use the information to help yourself to change your habits. You need to control unnecessary eating and foods that will undermine your weight loss.

Work is a dietary trigger for my wife. She is a physical therapist. Eating sweets is a profession-wide habit. It's funny, respiratory therapists smoke and physical therapists love sugar. Physical therapists will use any excuse to stock the department with cakes, candy, cookies or other sweets. ("It's Guy Fawkes day, did anyone bring cookies?") These snacks disappear without anyone "eating very much." If it weren't for her turbo-charged metabolism, my wife would be bigger than me. It is nothing to consume an extra 400 calories in a situation like that. You need to avoid eating when you are not hungry.

Wrigley Field is a trigger for many people here in Chicago. No sooner do you wedge your rear end into a bleacher seat than your subconscious mind whispers to you (several times), "Hot dog and beer." A hot dog and a beer have around 350 calories, none of which your body can put to good use.

There are a lot of triggers. Perhaps on dateless Saturday nights you rent old movies and eat chips (150 calories in an ounce of potato chips) and drink soda pop. Maybe you eat junk food in the car on a long trip. Watching a football game on TV can trigger you to eat pizza, corn doodles, pork rinds and other unnecessary calories. (We should re-name it foodball.)

Stress is also a trigger. Many of us eat when we are worried or emotionally upset. Try to take solace in some-thing other than food.

You need to recognize this behavior and change it. When you do your visualizing, picture your ideal self overcoming this behavior. You can visualize a picture (like a large poster or movie screen) of the behavior you want to change; then have your ideal self tear it to shreds.

⬜️ *Even if change doesn't come easy, keep trying and keep visualizing. Even a reduction in emotional eating will help.*

Eat Only At The Table

Don't wander around the house eating a bologna sandwich or snack in front of the television. If you eat anything, eat it at your kitchen table. This will cut down on nervous eating and will make you think before you eat. Snacking in front of the television isn't usually done out of hunger; it's done out of habit or from nervous eating.

Wait A Few Minutes
Before Taking Seconds

It takes a while for your body to realize that it is full. When you finish a meal and you are still hungry, wait 10 or 15 minutes before getting more food. After waiting, you may discover that you are not hungry. This is just another way for you to eat less without feeling deprived.

Eat Vegetarian One Day Each Week

It's a good way to limit your consumption of heavy foods that are hard to digest. It gives your digestive system a break and helps you clean out. Also vegetarian meals are usually low in calories. In general, it is better for you to eat low on the food chain. I agree with Jefferson (Thomas, not George) when he said that meat should be used as a condiment. Since a lot of the poison we dump in the environment ends up in animal fat, this is not a bad idea. On a cleaner planet, meat and dairy products would not be nearly as bad as they are here.

Leave The Table As Soon As You Are Finished

This may not be necessary for you, unless you are one of those people who can pick apart an entire turkey carcass and eat it during an after-dinner conversation. My sister is like that. If we don't get her away from the table, there won't be any leftovers for the next day. She can make an entire pie disappear, one small sliver at a time. (Apparently there are fewer calories in it if you take small pieces.)

This is another example of nervous eating. If it is one of your habits, just get away from the table. Start to take walks after dinner. That will be easier than trying to control your eating while sitting in front of a table full of food.

Don't Sample Foods While Cooking

This was always a problem for me. I love to cook and I'd always fix myself little snacks while I was cooking. My wife would come home and I'd already had the equivalent of two dinners and three desserts. But I never let that stop me from having more food. She hates to eat alone and I really didn't mind overeating — a man's got to do what a man's got to do.

I tried drinking a little wine, just so I wouldn't eat so much. After we put out the fire, we decided that wasn't such a good idea. I finally started chewing on carrot and celery sticks while cooking. It wasn't as much fun as the wine, but it was safer.

Eating while cooking is just another way to get extra calories. If you really have to have something while cooking, cut up some carrot and celery sticks. The calories are minimal and it will keep your mouth busy.

Don't Do Anything Else While Eating

A little snappy dinner conversation is all right, even encouraged. Talking will make you pause between bites and slow down. You may find that you are not only losing weight, but the members of your family are actually talking to each other. If you really want to cut down on your eating, invite someone over who you can't stand to listen to. It will make you want to get up from the table quickly.

▭ *When you eat, you should take time to chew, taste and enjoy your food. Don't read, work or watch TV. It will make you eat too quickly and absentmindedly, and you will consume more than you had intended.*

Control Yourself In Situations Where You Are Likely To Overeat

Exercise some control at parties and other events where you allow yourself to go off your program. Let's use the birthday as an example. Have a small piece of cake. Have ice cream, if you want it. Just don't overdo it. Your subconscious mind may be screaming to you, "Yeah, baby! Party time! Cake and ice cream! I'll start tomorrow!" Try to have a little control. It's one thing to allow yourself a food you do not normally eat. It's another to give yourself carte blanche. (You don't want to wake up in that gutter next to Ray Milland if you can avoid it.)

This was a hard thing for me to do at first. Once I'd given myself permission to eat incorrectly, I'd eat anything and everything. The poor host and hostess would have to make "food runs" during the party. The hostess would be shaking her head and mumbling to herself, "I could have sworn I fixed plenty of food." The host would be counting heads to make sure ten hungry stevedores hadn't crashed his party.

Don't save your appetite for a party. This is a tradition in my family. On Thanksgiving morning my mother will say, "Why do you want breakfast? We're eating a big meal at three." Skipping breakfast is a great way to ensure that you'll eat fast and you'll eat too much at dinner. The rules about blood sugar aren't suspended just because it's a holiday.

My weakness is pizza. When we order, I can just about finish a large one by myself. I still indulge myself with pizza once in a while, but I take a few steps to control my eating. I have a salad first and I eat very slowly, chewing it thoroughly. As a result, I eat about half as much as I used to, and I don't feel as if I'm sacrificing anything. Another way to save calories is to eat a vegetarian pizza. The worst things for you on a pizza are the greasy, processed meats.

My wife and I spent two weeks in Florida with her parents over the Christmas holidays. Her mother makes cookies that would make Mrs. Fields hang her head in shame. We were ready for a vacation of heavy eating and wonderful desserts. I lost three pounds over the holidays. Although the opportunity presented itself, I did not eat uncontrollably. I regulated my appetite by eating a lot of fruit. After dinner I'd promise myself a cookie only after eating a pear or an apple. After eating the fruit, the cookie was just not as appealing (although a few times eating fruit didn't stop me from having a cookie — they are really good). Since we were on vacation, I had plenty of time to go to the gym. I doubled the amount of time I spent working out and spent a lot of time golfing and swimming. Even though I consumed more food and ate more incorrectly than usual, I did manage to lose some weight.

So don't abandon all self-control when the opportunity presents itself. You can enjoy foods that you love on special occasions and still maintain your weight loss. I know it sounds like a broken record, but visualization will help you by giving you enough self-control so that every holiday is not a gustatory disaster.

E

Health Considerations

The majority of people will lose weight following the advice in this book. There will be a few people who will still have problems with either being able to follow the program or not getting the results they should have. Some will just not be able to control overeating. They will benefit from this section. Also contained here is information that will help you to feel better while losing weight even if you're not having any problems with your program.

Be Aware If You Have Digestive Problems

If you're a person who has cracked the windows in the car by belching or your family refuses to ride in a car with you after a meal or people say things to you like, "It's not the smell, it's the burning of my eyes," or you bought a dog just so you have someone to blame, this section is for you. Excess gas results from incomplete digestion or an imbalance in your bowel flora.

Listen To Your Body

If you have problems with digestion, they need to be addressed. These problems can contribute to food allergies, they can cause you to hold a lot of water weight and they can cause you to perpetually overeat. If digestive problems persist, they can completely undermine your efforts. If they're bad enough, you may be constantly fatigued or have other health problems.

Do you frequently have the following symptoms?

- Gas shortly after eating
- Gas one to four hours after eating
- Loss of desire for meat (not being a vegetarian for moral or other reasons, meat just doesn't appeal to you)
- Fatigue after meals
- Indigestion
- Constipation or diarrhea
- Bloating after meals
- Do not care to eat breakfast.

If you do, it is vital that you eat plenty of fruit and vegetables, stop eating sugar and enriched white flour, exercise, eat slowly, chew your food thoroughly and drink plenty of water. For most people, the problems with digestion will improve by doing these things. A few people will have problems that persist in spite of these changes.

Are There Any Benefits To Food Combining?

One popular solution to digestive problems and the weight problems they cause is food combining (or, more correctly, noncombining). Dr. Herbert Shelton wrote about this style of eating in the 1930s. It was made popular again by Judy Mazel and Susan Shultz in *The Beverly Hills Diet* and by Harvey and Marilyn Diamond in *Fit For Life*.

On this plan you eat fruit in the morning, grains and vegetables in the afternoon, and protein and vegetables in the evening. You never eat fruit with anything else and you never eat protein with starch. The argument is that your digestive system is so maladaptive that it doesn't handle different combinations of foods very well. There are different kinds of enzymes that work at different pHs to digest protein and starch.

In the Diamonds' book they want 70 percent of the food you eat to be fresh fruits and vegetables. (This part I agree with.) Eating in this fashion and paying attention to which combinations of foods you eat is fine. It will do you no harm. I know some people who follow this philosophy and claim great results. People with colitis often benefit from eating single-food meals. The problem is that it requires a great deal of discipline. Many people can't stay with it because their favorite food combinations are not allowed. You can't have a sandwich with meat or cheese in it. You can't have meat and potatoes. You can't have meat and cheese. You can't have cereal and fruit. You can't have fruit late in the day. It may well be a good program, but if you can't discipline yourself to follow it, it is useless.

The problem may not be that a combination of meat and starch is bad for your digestion, but rather that many people have digestive problems because they eat nothing but meat and starch, often too quickly, with little or no fresh vegetables and fruit.

I find that I function better if I do not have any heavy protein during the day. Protein is harder to digest than carbohydrates, and you spend a lot of energy digesting it. I find that I have much more energy during the day if I am not spending it digesting protein (or at least animal protein; legumes and other vegetable sources of protein do not seem to be as difficult).

You don't have to discipline yourself to eat food in certain combinations if you are thoroughly chewing your food, avoiding refined foods, drinking plenty of water and eating mostly fresh (preferably raw) fruits and vegetables. If your meals consist mostly of starch and protein and you eat too fast, don't be surprised if your digestion is not good.

I like to have oatmeal with fresh fruit in the morning, brown rice with protein at dinner and sometimes a little cheese on a salad (that I usually eat with a slice of whole grain bread). All of these things are not allowed by the doctrine of food combining. I don't think my digestive tract is so fragile that eating these combinations of foods is a problem.

Protein

If you have problems with digestion, most of your symptoms will improve just by cutting refined food out of your diet, chewing your food until it is liquid and eating a lot of fresh fruit and vegetables. Exercise will also help your digestion.

In your dietary diary see how much protein you are eating. You don't need very much, but most Americans don't feel like they've had a valid meal unless there is some sort of animal protein in it. According to the National Research Council, a 200-pound person needs between three and four ounces of protein per day. Four ounces of chuck steak has about 25 grams of protein, four ounces of white chicken meat has about 34 grams, one ounce of peanuts has about seven grams, and one cup of yogurt has about 12 grams of protein. Take your weight in pounds, divide it in half and that's about how much protein you need (in grams) per day.

$$\frac{\text{Weight (lbs.)}}{2} = \text{Protein (g.) per day}$$

It is easier on your digestive system if you do not get all of your protein from animal sources. One of the arguments against vegetarianism is that vegetables do not contain "complete" proteins. This means that vegetables do not have all of the essential amino acids.

Proteins are made up of amino acids which are small molecules. If a protein is a freight train, then an amino acid is one of the cars. There are 21 amino acids, eight of which are essential to your diet. An essential amino acid is one which the body cannot produce by itself. It must be provided by the diet.

Animal proteins have all of the essential amino acids; vegetable proteins usually do not. You can get all of your amino acids from vegetables, however, but you have to work a little to get them. Green leafy vegetables are good for you, but they are not a good source of protein. (This may be why so many "salad-bar" vegetarians seem so sickly.) If you eat vegetables for protein, you should get plenty of whole grains (like brown rice and whole wheat) and legumes (like nuts, peas and beans). One cup of peas has 8.1 grams of protein and one cup of brown rice has 4.8 grams of protein. The vegetable sources of protein are much easier to digest than the animal proteins.

What Your Body Needs To Digest Foods Properly

If you are chewing your food to liquid, not eating refined foods and getting plenty of fresh fruits and vegetables and your digestive problems persist, it is possible that you lack hydrochloric acid, normal bowel flora or digestive enzymes.

Perhaps you've taken antibiotics several times in your

life. Fighting an infection with antibiotics is a lot like hunting rabbits with high explosives. If you see the rabbit in a field and blow it up, you've also killed several squirrels, some birds and your cousin Alfred who was a bit too close to the little fellow. Antibiotics kill the bacteria involved with the infection, but they also kill bacteria that belong in your body, most notably the bacteria in your large intestine.

This is not to say that you should never use antibiotics. Under the right circumstances, they could save your life. They are valuable drugs and have saved many people from life-threatening infections. They have, however, been overused in the past and have sometimes been used irresponsibly for things like chronic acne and viral infections. (An antibiotic is useless against a virus, so don't bother your doctor for an antibiotic for your cold.)

Antibiotic therapy may cause yeast to proliferate in the intestines. This can lead to chronic yeast and bladder infections and possibly allergies. If you have been on antibiotics often in your life and you do not enjoy good health now, you may need supplementation with acidophilus and possibly some other things. Acidophilus is available in some supermarkets and most health food stores. It is a supplement designed to replace colon bacteria that have been killed after antibiotic therapy.

Betaine hydrochloride is also available in health food stores. It is a supplement for people who don't produce enough stomach acid to digest their food. A person who doesn't produce enough stomach acid may become bloated and/or fatigued after eating a meal (especially a meal that contains a lot of protein), may have allergies and may crave sweets. Sometimes he or she may have nausea or even a sensation of burning in the stomach. Be careful if you take betaine hydrochloride on an empty stomach or have a hiatal hernia, it can give you some pretty severe epigastric burning. It is best not to take betaine hydrochloride without the assistance of a health care professional. If you need it, betaine hydrochloride will help you digest protein. There are also digestive enzymes from vegetable sources that may be helpful. Sometimes removing certain foods (usually beef or dairy) will aid your digestion. As your diet improves, it will become more obvious which foods bother you.

Often gall bladder problems may make it difficult for you to digest fat. These are potentially serious and can give you severe pain under the bottom of the right side of the rib cage or in the right shoulder. Sometimes you will see a lot of "mucous" in your stool, which is really undigested fat. Pay careful attention to this because a gall bladder problem can lead to surgery and is potentially a medical emergency. If you suspect your gall bladder is a problem, you should consult your physician.

The Benefits Of Applied Kinesiology

It really isn't a good idea to diagnose and treat digestive problems on your own. I would recommend a health care professional who uses applied kinesiology. These are natural health care practitioners. Most are chiropractors, but some are osteopaths, medical doctors (allopaths) or dentists. In order to be in the International College of Applied Kinesiology (ICAK), one has to be a licensed health care professional and have taken classes in applied kinesiology beyond his or her professional degree. Be careful, there are a lot of unlicensed people doing some very strange things and calling it applied kinesiology. You can call the ICAK at 913-542-1801 to find a practitioner in your area.

It isn't that the ICAK has a monopoly on nutritional information; they're just one source. You may know of someone in your area or have a friend who can make a recommendation. The point is to get help from someone who knows what he or she is doing.

Be Aware Of The Possibility
Of Food Allergies

Chemicals In The Environment

Our bodies have been continually assaulted by chemicals. There's air pollution from internal combustion engines, production of electricity and factories. The pollution is washed into the ground by rain, then incorporated into the vegetables we eat. We dump pesticides on our crops. We inject the animals we eat with antibiotics and hormones. We put preservatives and colorings into our food.

The government determines "safe" levels of various pollutants and additives. Unfortunately no one has studied the cumulative effect all of these chemicals are having on us. We still have the bodies of poor dumb cave people and are not prepared for this chemical onslaught.

The result of ingesting these "safe" levels of chemicals is an increase in cancer. Also, have you noticed how many "new" diseases there are, such as "fibro myalgia," the "yuppie flu" or "chronic fatigue syndrome"? Another thing that has emerged with the poisoning of the planet and food supply is an increase in allergies. If you spend a lot of time not feeling very well, allergies are a definite possibility.

Identifying Allergic Reactions

The most common response I get when I suggest to a patient that he or she may be allergic to a certain food is, "Oh, I couldn't be allergic to that. I eat it all of the time." The image most people have of an allergic response is that of someone going into a sneezing fit or breaking out in hives when unknowingly eating something with an allergen in it.

Many, including a lot of doctors, think an allergic response is sudden, severe and obvious. It's actually more complicated than that.

Dr. Herbert Rinkel characterized three kinds of allergic reactions. The type of reaction we've been discussing is called a "fixed" reaction. It is the same every time you eat a food, even if it is only a small amount.

Another type of reaction is called a "cyclic" allergy. It is the type of allergy that doesn't bother a person unless he or she consumes a lot of the allergen or has it often. If you are allergic to dairy and you don't feel bad if you have a dairy product once or twice a week, that may not be enough to cause you to react. If you have it at three meals for a couple of days in a row, then you may have some problems. If a food bothers you when you eat it, but not all of the time, it is a cyclic allergy.

The third type of reaction is called an "addictive" allergy. It is the kind of allergy where the person has to have that particular food every day. He or she may have withdrawal symptoms if a meal with that food is missed.

Addictive Allergies

Spotting an addictive allergy can be tricky. If the food in question is corn, for instance, you can be eating corn and not realizing it. Most candy bars, ice cream, soda pop and other sweetened products contain corn sweetener. Corn starch is a common food additive and is frequently found in sauces made in restaurants. A person can be getting corn every day and not realize it.

Often a person with an addictive allergy will overeat chronically or be obese. It is the one thing that can make your efforts in this book go for nothing. If you are a compulsive eater, or you absolutely have to have chocolate, a can of soda, potato chips or some such food every day, you may have an addictive allergy to one or more foods. This is the thing to suspect when someone is a "junk food junkie." It's like being an alcoholic.

Theron Randolph called alcoholism the ultimate food allergy. I strongly recommend you get his book, *An Alternative Approach To Allergies*.

Many people are allergic to additives and pesticides. Often they find that they can eat organically grown versions of foods that otherwise might bother them. Chemical allergies are a common problem. Many times people will think all fruit bothers them, when in reality it is the pesticide sprayed on the fruit.

Allergies can be responsible for a wide variety of symptoms such as:

- skin problems
- headaches
- fatigue
- blurred vision
- arthritis
- digestive problems
- asthma
- muscle weakness
- mental disorders such as mood swings
- depression and even schizophrenia.

In fact there are few symptoms that can't be caused by allergies. Two symptoms that are common to allergy sufferers are obesity and the tendency to overeat. There is even strong evidence to suggest that gallstones are caused by food allergy.

Frequently an allergy sufferer will be written off by his or her doctors as a hypochondriac. The patient will often have a lot of bizarre and seemingly unrelated symptoms. They may have headaches, nausea, arthritic pains, insomnia, skin problems or even mental disorders. Tests are performed, but seldom is a disease process identified. Often doctors indulge themselves in the ultimate medical conceit, "If I can't find it, it must be in your head."

One way to tell if you've ingested a food to which you're allergic is if your pulse speeds up. Some people are so allergic to certain foods, it feels as if their heart is pounding in their neck or head after a meal. If your pulse increases by ten beats per minute or more after eating, you may be allergic to something that you've eaten. This doesn't happen to everyone with food allergies, but if your pulse does speed up after eating, you probably have a food allergy.

If you cannot control your eating, or if you try to give up junk food and become sick, you may have an addictive allergy. If you are extremely obese and nothing seems to be working for you in your effort to lose weight, you may have some food allergies.

Food Allergies And Rotation Diets

You can have some allergies and not be as sick and miserable as I've described. Frequently patients see me and are in reasonably good shape, even exercise regularly, but are unable to reach their ideal weight. I've seen people who run triathlons who are unable to get rid of the last little bit of a pot belly. Frequently they are allergic to a favorite food. They will often lose as much as 10 pounds by removing wheat, dairy or some other allergen from their diet. Often their athletic performance improves as well.

The most common allergens are corn, wheat, yeast, eggs, beef, soy and citrus. Diet programs have addressed these in the past. The most recent is *The Berger Diet.*

Dr. Berger's program consists of cleaning out from the seven allergens listed here, followed by a rotation diet. Dr. Berger has all of the foods and recipes laid out for you. It will work pretty well if your allergies are confined to one of these seven substances. It is a difficult diet to follow but not because of hunger. You're allowed to eat as much as you want. But the food is sometimes difficult to get and prepare.

The idea is to avoid the food you are allergic to for a few weeks. After a period of avoidance, the food is not to be eaten more than every four or five days. If you are not sure of the foods you are allergic to, or if you are allergic to many different foods, there are general rotation diets. With these you don't eat the same food or food from a member of the same biological family (for instance, tomatoes and green peppers are related) more than every four days.

You must be careful. If you have an addictive allergy, you may go through withdrawal symptoms while giving up the food. Expect not to feel good for a few days. Sometimes reintroducing the food after abstinence will cause you to react severely to it. It is best to read and learn more about allergies and to get professional help if you need it.

It is not in the scope of this book to tell you how to identify your food allergies and what to do about them. Often in the office patients will respond very well to removal of the offending food, then reintroducing it after some time (on a rotation basis) and giving them certain nutrients. Many people with allergies respond very well to chiropractic adjustments.

Don't rely on most doctors to understand a proper approach to allergies. The skin tests traditionally used to identify allergies are not very accurate. (The tests are as much as 80 percent inaccurate according to Dr. Marshall Mandell.)

There are a group of physicians who practice environmental medicine. You can contact the American Academy of Environmental Medicine at: (303) 622-9755 to find a practitioner in your area. If allergies are a problem, you owe it to yourself to learn about them and seek proper help. There are some books on the subject that you will find helpful:

- *An Alternative Approach to Allergies* by Theron Randolph, M.D.
- *Brain Allergies* by William Philpott, M.D.
- *Dr. Mandell's 5-Day Allergy Relief System* by Marshall Mandell, M.D.

Get Help If You Need It

Following what is written in this book will work for most people. You just need to make the effort. Contained here is a way to lose weight without being hungry, a way that will make most people have a great deal of energy and get healthy while enjoying the process. Even a lot of people suffering from allergies and digestive problems will improve by cleaning up their diets and by exercising.

Everyone who reads this is different. I don't know your situation, physical condition or the kinds of health problems you may have. You may try very hard to apply what is written here and not do well. You may need help with a health problem that hasn't been mentioned. You may need a support group, such as Overeaters Anonymous. You may need help with motivation. If you are not successful on your own, by all means, get help.

Perhaps you have trouble motivating yourself to exercise. You may do better if you go to a structured exercise class or even get a personal trainer. You may have a physical problem that needs attention, such as allergies, digestive disorders or even an underactive thyroid. Whatever your problem, if you're not succeeding on your own, please get help.

Very often obese individuals have problems with self-image. Sometimes there is a history of abuse early in life. Some people won't be able to succeed without some sort of counseling or support group. If you fall into this group, please get the help you need.

Some individuals are so obese that their condition is life-threatening. A medically supervised program may be in order. Try to find a doctor or a program that will emphasize exercise and education about food, and has counseling or counseling some sort of support group. It should be a holistic program. Your doctor should pay attention to thyroid function and other potential health problems, not just take the attitude, "Drink this slop and call me in the morning." A liquid diet may be necessary in an extreme situation, where being obese is actually more dangerous than going on a drastic program but not when it's a case of, "Gee, Doc, I want to be thin and pretty in a hurry."

▭ *No matter what kind of shape you are in, you should get a thorough physical examination before starting your program. There is a possibility that your weight problem is caused by hypothyroidism or some other health problem. You can also discuss with your doctor the type of exercise program you are planning.*

Expect To Feel Good

One of the worst things about getting fat is feeling tired and miserable. Exercising and eating right will make most people feel great, even if they are still overweight. Expect to feel good. That should be your real goal.

If you've been eating a lot of sweets and refined carbohydrates for a long time, you may need to supplement yourself with vitamin B and probably a multimineral. If you are really out of shape, you may have a lot of aches and pains that will keep you from wanting to exercise. I recommend a good chiropractor. (I know it sounds prejudiced, but it's my book and I can say what I want.) Most chiropractors have a good background in nutrition, so if you need supplementation, your chiropractor could be a good source of nutritional information.

We've discussed exercising from the standpoint of getting your heart rate up and burning calories. There are two other kinds of exercises you should do. Yoga will help you with flexibility. Exercising with weights or resistance will tone your muscles. You will become stronger and your body will take on a shape that you'll be proud of. Weight lifting will also increase your lean body mass, which will cause you to burn more calories in your day-to-day life. Deep breathing will increase your energy by increasing tissue oxygenation and the removal of cellular waste by the lymphatic system. Try taking a slow deep breath and holding it for about 30 seconds, then let it out very slowly (exhale for about twice as long as you inhale). Doing ten breaths like this will increase your energy almost immediately.

If you are the kind of person who can look at food and gain weight, you may have a very slow metabolism. You may be very tired and have trouble following through. The breathing exercises will help you. Exercising in a cool room will help you increase your metabolism, as will taking a cold shower or finishing a shower with cold water. Taking a sauna followed by a cold shower will also help stimulate your metabolism. Certain supplements will aid in stimulating your sympathetic nervous system, such as vitamin B, carnitine (an amino acid), and essential fatty acids. If your metabolism is slow, you may need the help of a chiropractor, especially one who uses applied kinesiology, to help stimulate your sympathetic nervous system.

If you have been eating a lot of junk food and you give it up, there is a possibility that you won't feel well at first. Be patient and don't give up. You should feel better after a few days.

Drink Water

Drink between six and eight 8-ounce glasses of water each day. Water enables you to eliminate waste. Many people think we urinate to get rid of water. That isn't the case. We lose more water from respiration. Your body spends water, which is precious to it, in order to get rid of small amounts of solid waste.

If your program is successful, you will begin breaking down fat. When fat breaks down, it creates waste products known as ketone bodies. These are eliminated by the kidneys, which need water to remove them. If you don't get enough water when you're losing weight, these waste products are not properly removed. You will feel tired and maybe even a little headachy.

One common complaint I get from patients when they're told to drink this much water is, "If I drank that much water, I'd live in the bathroom." That's a sure sign that you need water. It means that your body is holding on to its waste until you provide it with enough water to get rid of some. You drink a little water and your body says, "Goody, I can get rid of some of this junk." And you have to go to the bathroom.

As you drink more water and your body becomes more hydrated, you will go to the bathroom less. This happens because you hold on to less of your body's wastes when you are well hydrated. Very often sinus problems improve in people who begin drinking water. Constipation is commonly present in people who do not drink enough water. Tea, milk, coffee, juice and other liquids don't count. You can drink these, but make sure you get the eight glasses of water.

What Kind Of Water Is Best?

There is a lot of controversy about which kind of water is the best to drink. Long ago, well and spring water were clean. They were rich in iron, calcium and other minerals. Today much of the water is polluted with pesticides and industrial waste. Every so often you hear of an inordinate number of people in the same area dying of cancer. Often hidden pollutants in the water are to blame. There are labs that will test your water and there are kits you can purchase to test for various pollutants at home. National Testing Lab, Inc. in Cleveland, Ohio, will test your water for heavy metals, pesticides and other contaminants for a modest fee. Their phone number is 1-800-458-3330. Locally we have a company called Environmental Management and Field Testing, in Evanston. They not only will test water, but they come to homes and test for mold, formaldehyde, lead, insecticides and other pollutants. Their phone number is 708-475-3696.

If you have a well, it is probably a good idea to filter the water from it. There are activated carbon and reverse osmosis filters available. This is an oversimplification but activated carbon is good for removing organic materials such as chemicals and pesticides. Reverse osmosis filters are good for removing metals such as lead and mercury. There are also filters that combine reverse osmosis and activated carbon. Make sure you change the filtering element when you're supposed to. Otherwise you may be adding pollutants to your drinking water.

There is a nonprofit organization that rates water filters called the National Sanitation Foundation (NSF). They certify filters and rate their effectiveness for removing specific pollutants from the water. They can be reached at:

P.O. Box 1468

Ann Arbor, Michigan 48106

When choosing a water filter, you can have your water tested, then choose the appropriate NSF-rated filter. If the filter you want to buy does not have an NSF rating, you can have the water tested before and after filtration.

Some people buy bottled distilled water. Proponents of distilled water claim that it is relatively pollution free. Critics say that it has no minerals and is not natural. If you place a cell into distilled water, it will explode. Another problem is that volatile pollutants (with a lower boiling point than water) can get distilled right in with the water.

City tap water has a lot of chlorine and fluorine in it. You cannot be completely sure that all of the contaminants have been removed. You should at least filter it.

There is bottled spring water for sale. Some of it is good, some of it is not. There are no controls over the quality of bottled water. You could start your own bottled water company with your tap and some jugs.

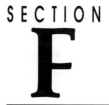

Miscellaneous

Here are some extra hints to help you achieve your goal, and to keep this book from being called *48 Ways To Lose Your Blubber.*

Avoid Common Mistakes

You will be able to see these on the David Letterman show under the heading "Stupid Dieter Tricks."

1. *Going on a half diet:* Trying to watch your weight during the day by undereating, but doing it without any real plan. Skipping breakfast, having a salad for lunch, etc. You're pretty proud of yourself and hardly notice that you had a can of Pepsi or a few chocolate chip cookies during the late afternoon. All you will accomplish by doing this is to begin a yo-yo dieting pattern and slow down your metabolism.

2. *Starting the day with donuts and coffee:* You're just starting your program and you've decided that you don't want to give up sweets just yet. Starting the day with sugar will screw up your eating pattern for the rest of the day. Eating nothing but sugar in the morning will make it very difficult to give up sugar because a few hours after this sugary breakfast your blood sugar will drop and you will crave sugar again. Make sure you eat a good (sugar-free) breakfast. If you don't want to give up sweets yet, it is better to have them in the form of dessert after a meal. Don't have sugar on an empty stomach. If you do not like to eat breakfast, you could be having problems digesting last night's dinner. If that is the case, eat fresh fruit in the morning and continue to eat fruit every two hours until you have lunch.

3. *Taking over-the-counter appetite suppressants:* Have you learned nothing?

4. *Having protein drinks for a meal:* I just went to the grocery store to see what the label on a popular brand says. Other than the fact that I'll need to finish my masters in chemistry to understand it, the stuff has both aspartame and sugar in it. Calling it food is really stretching the definition. Eat food. There is really nothing wrong with that. You need to eat. Enjoy eating. Just be selective about what you eat. If you use some common sense and exercise, there is no reason to subject yourself to a program like this.

There is a liquid diet program available to chiropractors called Ultra Balance. I found it to be superior to many similar programs. The person dieting is required to have seven cups of vegetables per day, there is a fiber source in the drink, there are no chemicals and it is hypoallergenic. The program requires you to exercise for 20 minutes per day. The manufacturer provides tapes, recipes (because you don't stay on the total liquid diet for more than a week). People who tried this lost weight quickly. Many I personally know of didn't keep it off. After all, it is a diet and the dieter is fed less food than his or her body needs. It is a very low-calorie program. For many the maintenance was harder than the dieting and they regained the weight.

5. *Exercising a body part that hurts:* Don't think that the pain will just go away. You may be courting a serious injury that will keep you from exercising. Change your exercise. If your knees hurt, start rowing instead of bicycling. If your shoulder hurts, bicycle instead of row. If the problem persists, see a physician.

6. *Eating a boring diet:* Just because you've given up eating many of your favorite junk foods doesn't mean you have to burn out on carrot and celery sticks. Healthy food can be enjoyable. Vary your foods. Approach this with a sense of discovery. Take time to find a variety of healthy foods that you like. Many ethnic cuisines, such as Middle Eastern and Oriental are healthy *and* enjoyable.

7. *Using aspartame:* I know I've mentioned aspartame (Nutra-Sweet) before, but this stuff is bad enough that it is worth mentioning again. From a dieter's standpoint, aspartame may be of no help to you in losing weight. It has fewer calories, but some physicians believe that it interferes with your body's mechanism for feeling full after a meal. It may actually contribute to overeating. You may not be worried about the increased chance of getting a brain tumor but the possibility of actually gaining weight may make you stay away from it.

8. *Drinking too much alcohol:* You wake up in the morning feeling like General Schwarzkopf and the boys are holding desert maneuvers on your tongue. You hear an ear-shattering noise that makes your head explode in pain. It's your wife opening the mail. Someone is playing the Anvil Chorus on your head. It's time for your morning exercise, so you jump right up and do it. (Right, and the check is in the mail, I'm from the government and I'm here to help you, and we can't print the third one.)

   A shot of whiskey or a glass of dry wine has about 80 calories, and 12 ounces of beer has about 150 calories. A six pack of beer has about 900 calories. A good bender is worth anywhere from 600 calories for a good buzz to a couple of thousand calories for an all-out drunken orgy. This isn't counting the junk food you may eat when your judgment is impaired.

9. *Becoming complacent:* Start to change your habits, begin to get some results and then allow yourself to plateau without reaching your goal. I don't know why this happens but often someone will lose ten pounds and be so thrilled with the results that they quit trying to lose anymore. Don't get complacent. It's all right to plateau for a little while and not try as hard to lose weight, but you should at least try to maintain your weight loss. Keep interested in the idea of losing weight and keep track of your weight. Think of it as a little vacation from your program, but keep your goal in mind. It will be easier to start in earnest if you

haven't gained back all of your weight during your hiatus.

10. *Using lack of time as an excuse:* Time is the most common excuse we use to keep from doing things we do not want to do. Not having time to shop for good foods, clean vegetables, cook healthy meals or exercise is usually not the problem. The problem is desire and willingness to make the effort to change. It would be best if you worked out 30 minutes per day. If you just work out for 15 minutes each day, you will still notice some improvement. Surely you can find 15 minutes to do some exercise. If it were sex, you'd find the time. The problem isn't time, it's motivation.

Visualizing takes a little bit of time each day, but you can do it while you do other things. Visualize during your workout, on your way to work or in the bathroom.

Usually excuses come in groups. I don't have time, I don't know what to do, my feet hurt, I'm tired and I really should wait until I'm ready (yes, that mythical time when my life is in order).

Frozen dinners, canned food and packaged mixes sell very well because people don't have time to cook. Please don't use time as an excuse to consume chemicals, hydrogenated fat and devitalized food. There are cookbooks written for busy people. Fresh vegetables take almost no time to prepare because they can be eaten raw. Many supermarkets now have salad bars. There are lots of meals you can make that take about as much time as a frozen dinner.

Cooking In A Hurry

I'm no Frugal Gourmet, but I do some cooking. My wife and I both work and we don't spend a lot of time in the kitchen (which is one reason we got into the habit of ordering carry-out food in the first place). Here are some things we make when we are in a hurry.

Chopped Salad

This one is easy. Take any vegetables that you have and put them in a food processor and chop them to a fine consistency. Use oil and vinegar as a dressing (or some people like other light dressings, like honey mustard or Caesar). It's very good for people who don't care much for vegetables and it's a great way to get rid of leftover vegetables. You can make extra for dinner and have some for lunch and dinner the next day. It only takes a couple of minutes to make.

Casseroles

Take any kind of meat and put it in a casserole dish. Add in a half cup of sherry and a half cup of bouillon. Slice vegetables and potatoes. Cover the casserole dish and bake at 375 degrees for about 35 minutes per pound. Some of the combinations we often use are:

- Chicken, pineapple, onions, garlic (two crushed cloves) seasoned with ginger and some of the juice from the pineapple.
- Chuck roast, onions, carrot, celery, red peppers, seasoned with salt and pepper.
- Chicken with julienne cut carrots and zucchini seasoned with ginger, soy sauce and garlic.
- Pork roast in red vermouth and beef bouillon. (Let this sit overnight. It is much better with organic pork.)
- Chicken with potatoes, carrots, onions, red pepper and a can of Progresso minestrone soup.
- Pork with pineapple.
- Beef with broccoli, cauliflower, carrots and potatoes.

You really don't need me to tell you what to put in your casserole dish. The more vegetables you use, the fewer you will have to prepare separately. Use seasoning and vegetables that you like. This is not gourmet cooking here. It's just a way to get away from frozen dinners without spending a lot of time cooking. These meals may spend an hour in the oven, but so do many TV dinners. The time spent putting the food in the casserole is minimal and can even be done in the morning or the previous evening.

Brown rice makes an excellent side dish. (Just a hint: use chicken or beef broth for half of the liquid and use about 25 percent more liquid than the directions tell you; you can drain the excess liquid and you won't burn the rice.) You can chop tomato, onion and green pepper into the brown rice before you cook it. Served with peas or green beans, it's a very nutritious meal.

Stir Frying

Stir frying is easy and fast. You use peanut oil with about a teaspoon of sesame oil. You partially cook any meat in the oil. Take the meat out and cook the vegetables over a hot flame for a short period of time (or don't use meat, there are many excellent vegetarian dishes). Season with soy sauce (sometimes thickened with a little arrowroot), garlic and ginger. There are a hundred books with stir-fry recipes. Most of the dishes are easy and quick to prepare.

Soups and Salads

Salads are quick to make, and with the right ingredients, make a complete meal. Soups are also easy to make and can provide meals for several days.

Eat Right Even If You're Busy

There are many good recipes that are quick and easy to make. There are many cookbooks that are written for people who are short of time. With a little effort you won't be living on Hamburger Helper, frozen dinners, canned foods and carry-out pizza anymore.

Busy people often use the fact that they have to eat in restaurants as an excuse for eating poorly. The other day I accepted a ride in my office manager's car. There was a fast-food bag on the floor and she offered an explanation (perhaps I've been a bit insufferable as a reformed junk food junkie). She said that she had had a very hectic day and just grabbed a hamburger, fries and a coke for lunch. Fearing that I may have been giving a few too many fire-and-brimstone speeches on the subject of nutrition, I didn't tell her that her fast-food eatery has salads (as do most burger chains now).

Restaurants are triggers. You may think of fast-food and your desire for grease is triggered. So, of course, you have a Big Mac and fries (a little over 600 empty calories and a lot of fat). The fact that you didn't have a salad has nothing to do with how much time you have. You could even have a small hamburger with the salad as a compromise to your grease craving. Many of my patients lament that they are unable to watch closely what they eat because they are busy and eat out frequently. They blame their love handles and pot bellies on business lunches. Just because you go to "Luigi's" for lunch doesn't mean that you have to stuff your face with linguini and garlic bread.

You're not fat because you're incapable of staying on a 1,200-calorie diet long enough to lose the weight. You're fat because you make too many fat decisions: that extra 150 calories because you really wanted a can of pop, the grease orgy at the hamburger stand or the sweets you feel you need at night while watching TV. You're fat because you are not active enough. You can use time as an excuse, but it won't make you thin. Take the time, lose the weight and you too can become insufferable.

Design Your Own Program

There it is, everything you wanted to know about losing weight, but were afraid to ask. The hardest part will be getting started. I know. I wore out a couch and three sets of batteries for the remote control saying, "I'll start tomorrow."

Take two weeks and write down what you eat every day. It may shock you into action. Set your goal and begin visualizing. If you keep track of what you're doing and visualize what you want to do, bingo! you've started.

Exercise is more important than any of the dietary changes. A decent half-hour workout will burn between 300 and 400 calories per day. That translates to 30 pounds per year. Exercise is especially important if you are the type of person who doesn't eat much but still can't lose weight.

When planning your program there are two considerations you should have. Which items involve the least amount of sacrifice and are easiest to do and which items will help you to lose the most weight. Things like chewing your food thoroughly, taking small portions and not taking seconds don't take much discipline. Maybe giving up sugar would not be a big deal for you. Make the changes that come easily to you right away.

It would be helpful for you to identify which changes will give you the most results. If you eat a lot of junk food, eating fruits and vegetables and controlling your blood sugar will be important, as will identifying any food allergies you may have. If you have digestive problems, you will need to bring those under control, usually by eating slowly and removing certain foods from your diet. Eat less dairy and animal protein.

A person who has no problem with digestion but can't seem to lose weight in spite of eating very little needs to be more active. The more exercise the better. Controlling eating habits is not as important for such a person (although it is not completely unimportant).

Just to give you an idea: The average American consumes between 2,000 and 3,000 calories per day. Count what you now eat and see if you are in that ballpark. If you are eating over 3,000 calories per day, your approach will be different from someone who consumes less than 2,000 calories per day. The person eating too much needs to bring that eating under control, but not by self-denial. You now possess the tools to cut down on your eating without starving yourself.

The person who eats very little needs to stimulate his or her metabolism. Exercise and eating plenty of fresh fruits and vegetables will help. Activity is the key for the person with a slow metabolism. If this is your problem, you need to be active at every opportunity. Think of the daily exercise as just a start.

⬜▭ *No matter how heavy you are, or what your reason for getting that way, all 50 ways will help you. Do as many of them as you can. Start with what comes easily to you, but always strive to change your bad habits for good ones. Remember you are a unique individual and your weight problem is also unique. Your scale will tell you how successful you are. If you plateau, add a new discipline or consider if you need to change what you eat. Consistent effort will pay off and you will be as thin as you want to be — permanently.*

Now What?

The last thing I want to do here is to create a dogma to be followed with blind obedience, like so many other diet and fitness books do. Think of this part as suggestions of how to apply the information that you have just read. There are 50 ways to lose your blubber, but some will serve you better than others. You need to know which disciplines are priorities. Much of the material is designed to help you develop discipline or requires none at all. The categories with an asterisk (*) next to them require discipline and are important. They are the key to your losing weight. It should also be mentioned here that if digestion or allergies are a problem, getting them taken care of is a top priority.

Here is a list of the 50 sections in this book:

1. Read This Book
2. Lose The Guilt
*3. Set Goals
*4. Visualize
5. Enjoy The Process
6. Keep A Food Diary
7. Lose Weight With A Friend
8. Avoid "All-Or-Nothing" Thinking
9. Don't Be In A Hurry
10. Reward Yourself
11. Take This One Day At A Time
12. You Don't "Have To" Do Anything
13. Don't Get Hung Up On Your Day-To-Day Weight
14. Keep Trying, Even Though You Feel As If You've Failed
15. Keep Trying, Even Though You Feel As If You've Succeeded
*16. Exercise, Exercise, Exercise
*17. Make Yourself Work Harder
18. Destroy Your Television
*19. Get Busy, Stop Being Sedentary
20. Don't Diet Or Get Hung Up On Calories
*21. Absolutely Avoid Refined Sugar
*22. Don't Starve Yourself
23. Eat If You're Hungry
*24. Eat Whole Grains
25. Don't Get Hung Up On Nutritional Fads And Buzz Words
26. Learn How To Read Labels And Choose Your Food
*27. Eat Lots Of Fresh Fruit And Vegetables
*28. Absolutely Avoid Commercially Fried Foods

*29. Buy Organically Grown Foods Whenever Possible
30. Learn To Control Cravings
*31. Eat Slowly. Chew Your Food Thoroughly
32. Learn To Like Plain Foods
33. Don't Clean Your Plate
34. Don't Clean Someone Else's Plate
35. Don't Eat If You're Not Hungry
36. Beware Of Triggers
37. Eat Only At The Table
38. Wait A Few Minutes Before Taking Seconds
39. Eat Vegetarian One Day Each Week
40. Leave The Table As Soon As You Are Finished
41. Don't Sample Foods While Cooking
42. Don't Do Anything Else While Eating
43. Control Yourself In Situations Where You Are Likely
    To Overeat
44. Be Aware If You Have Digestive Problems
45. Be Aware Of The Possibility Of Food Allergies
46. Get Help If You Need It
47. Expect To Feel Good
48. Drink Water
49. Avoid Common Mistakes
50. Design Your Own Program

The key to your weight-loss program is to control the quality of the food you eat and to increase your activity level. The more successful you are at those two things, the more successful you will be at losing weight.

Perhaps as you read this, the thought of giving up sugar or fried food is unthinkable, or you don't feel that you have time to exercise. *You must make it your goal to implement these changes.* Visualizing will help you to change. I can't stress that enough.

Just because there are 12 "have tos" listed here doesn't mean there is not room for individual variation. I have a patient who has been fairly successful with his program, but he likes to have a cookie with his lunch. There are certain meals that I like to have French bread with and occasionally I like pasta. Eating cookies, pasta and French bread will interfere with anyone's attempt to lose weight. But if you are willing to be strict in other areas, you can indulge yourself in the things you really love. If you are being too indulgent, don't worry, the scale will tell you. If you are not losing weight, just start being a little stricter.

Everyone is different. Some people will have a lot of trouble giving up certain foods, but will love to exercise. Others will be able to control the quality of their foods, but will want to exercise minimally.

You will have to adapt your program to your own circumstances. For instance, people who travel a lot have special problems following a routine. You just have to take it one day at a time. Each day will present you with choices. If you have time to kill at the airport, touring the facility with a brisk walk will serve you better than time spent in the cocktail lounge looking at your watch. People often complain about airplane food. You can order vegetarian meals or bring fresh fruit and vegetables with you. You can choose hotels with health clubs or swimming pools. There are more and more of them — we're in the middle of a fitness craze. If you can't get a hotel with a health club, perhaps you can get one that is several stories tall. Get a room near the top and use the stairs.

As bad as diet soda is for you, the concept that makes it sell is a good one. If you drink a can of soda, it's about 150 extra calories. A diet drink saves you 149 calories. Don't do this, drink water and save the full 150 calories. Throughout the day there are decisions you make that will either help or hinder your weight loss. Deciding whether to walk or to drive someplace, deciding whether to have a salad or a hamburger for lunch, or deciding whether to snack on carrots or potato chips are the types of decisions that will determine your success or failure. By burning off an extra 100 calories when the opportunity presents itself and by choosing food that will nourish you and not just add empty calories consistently every day will help you lose weight and feel better.

During your program, you may notice that at different times, your resolve varies. I had been very strict with myself for the first 20 pounds. I exercised more than I had to and I was very strict about what I ate. When I broke the 20-pound barrier, I began exercising less and eating more. For about three weeks I didn't lose anything. (For what it's worth, I didn't gain anything either.) After the three weeks I became more interested in exercise again and started to lose weight. You will experience similar highs and lows. Don't worry too much about them. *Remember, you are trying for permanent change and good health. The weight loss will really just be a pleasant side effect.*

CRAVINGS

This is by no means a complete chart of all causes of cravings. It includes some of the more common ones and some of the cravings that will keep you from losing weight. It must also be understood that food allergies may cause food cravings and the tendency to overeat.

Craving	Reason	Symptoms	Solution
Sugar	Low blood sugar	• Tired and irritable if meals are missed	• Eat every 2 hours • Avoid sugar and white flour
Sugar	Poor digestion	• Bloating and fatigue after meals • Gas or indigestion • Loss of desire for meat	• Eat slowly and chew food well • Eat fresh, raw fruit and vegetables • May need betaine HCl or digestive supplements
Fried food Greasy food Chocolate Meat and dairy	Lack of essential fatty acids	• Dry skin • Itching • Muscle fatigue and soreness	• Eat legumes or avocados • Supplement with black currant oil or flax seed oil • Avoid fried food and hydrogenated oil
General overeating	Poor digestion and absorption	• Gas, bloating • Eats but doesn't seem to be satisfied	• Betaine HCl, digestive enzymes • Eat slowly and chew food well • Eat fresh, raw fruits and vegetables
General overeating	Poor nutrition (eating too many empty calories)		• Eat lots of fresh fruits and vegetables, whole grains — "cave man diet" • May need supplements
Salt	Functional adrenal deficiency	• Fatigue • Hard to get up in the morning • May have knee or low back pain	• Strict avoidance of sugar and white flour • Eat every 2 hours • May need supplement

Bibliography

Conrad Levinson, Jay. **Guerrilla Marketing Attack.** Houghton Mifflin, Co., Boston, MA: 1989.

Erasmus, Udo. **Fats And Oils.** Alive Books, Vancouver, Canada: 1986.

Golding, Lawrence A., et al. **The Y's Way To Physical Fitness.** Published for YMCA by Human Kinetics Publishers, Inc., Champaign, IL: 1982.

Mandell, Marshall Dr., and Randolph, Theron G., **Dr. Mandell's Five-Day Allergy Relief System.** Harper & Row, New York, NY: 1988.

McArdle, William, Katch, Frank and Katch, Victor. **Exercise Physiology,** 3rd Ed. Lea and Febiger, Philadelphia, PA: 1991.

Pennington, Jean A.T., and Nichols Church, Helen. **Food Values.** Harper & Row, New York, NY: 1985.

Philpott, William, M.D., and Kalita, Dwight, Ph.D. **Brain Allergies: The Psycho-Nutrient Connection.** Keats Publishing, New Canaan, CT: 1987.

Randolph, Theron, G., M.D. and Moss, Ralph W. **An Alternative Approach To Allergies.** Harper & Row, New York, NY: 1980.

Steinman, David. **Diet For A Poisoned Planet: How To Choose Safe Food For You & Your Family.** Crown Publishers, Inc., New York, NY: 1990.

Winter, Ruth. **A Consumer's Dictionary Of Food Additives.** New Revised Ed. Crown Publishers, Inc., New York, NY: 1984.

New Books . . .
from Health Communications

HEAL YOUR SELF-ESTEEM: Recovery From Addictive Thinking
Bryan Robinson, Ph.D.

Do you have low self-esteem? Do you blame others for your own unhappiness? If so, you may be an addictive thinker. The 10 Principles For Healing, an innovative, positive approach to recovery, are integrated into this book to provide a new attitude with simple techniques for recovery.

ISBN 1-55874-119-4   **$9.95**

HEALING ENERGY: The Power Of Recovery
Ruth Fishel, M.Ed., C.A.C.

Linking the newest medical discoveries in mind/body/spirit connections with the field of recovery, this book illustrates how to balance ourselves mentally, physically and spiritually to overcome our addictive behavior.

ISBN 1-55874-128-3   **$9.95**

CREDIT, CASH AND CO-DEPENDENCY: The Money Connection
Yvonne Kaye, Ph.D.

Co-dependents and Adult Children seem to experience more problems than most as money can be used as an anesthetic or fantasy. Yvonne Kaye writes of the particular problems the co-dependent has with money, sharing her own experiences.

ISBN 1-55874-133-X   **$9.95**

THE LAUNDRY LIST: The ACoA Experience
Tony A. and Dan F.

Potentially The Big Book of ACoA, *The Laundry List* includes stories, history and helpful information for the Adult Child of an alcoholic. Tony A. discusses what it means to be an ACoA and what the self-help group can do for its members.

ISBN 1-55874-105-4   **$9.95**

LEARNING TO SAY NO: Establishing Healthy Boundaries
Carla Wills-Brandon, M.A.

If you grew up in a dysfunctional family, establishing boundaries is a difficult and risky decision. Where do you draw the line? Learn to recognize yourself as an individual who has the power to say no.

ISBN 1-55874-087-2   **$8.95**

3201 S.W. 15th Street,
Deerfield Beach, FL 33442-8190
1-800-441-5569

Health Communications, Inc.®

Other Books By . . .
Health Communications

ADULT CHILDREN OF ALCOHOLICS (Expanded)
Janet Woititz

Over a year on *The New York Times* Best-Seller list, this book is the primer on Adult Children of Alcoholics.

ISBN 1-55874-112-7   **$8.95**

STRUGGLE FOR INTIMACY
Janet Woititz

Another best-seller, this book gives insightful advice on learning to love more fully.

ISBN 0-932194-25-7   **$6.95**

BRADSHAW ON: THE FAMILY: A Revolutionary Way of Self-Discovery
John Bradshaw

The host of the nationally televised series of the same name shows us how families can be healed and individuals can realize full potential.

ISBN 0-932194-54-0   **$9.95**

HEALING THE SHAME THAT BINDS YOU
John Bradshaw

This important book shows how toxic shame is the core problem in our compulsions and offers new techniques of recovery vital to all of us.

ISBN 0-932194-86-9   **$9.95**

*HEALING THE CHILD WITHIN: Discovery and Recovery for
Adult Children of Dysfunctional Families* — Charles Whitfield, M.D.

Dr. Whitfield defines, describes and discovers how we can reach our Child Within to heal and nurture our woundedness.

ISBN 0-932194-40-0   **$8.95**

A GIFT TO MYSELF: A Personal Guide To Healing My Child Within
Charles L. Whitfield, M.D.

Dr. Whitfield provides practical guidelines and methods to work through the pain and confusion of being an Adult Child of a dysfunctional family.

ISBN 1-55874-042-2   **$11.95**

*HEALING TOGETHER: A Guide To Intimacy And Recovery For
Co-dependent Couples* — Wayne Kritsberg, M.A.

This is a practical book that tells the reader why he or she gets into dysfunctional and painful relationships, and then gives a concrete course of action on how to move the relationship toward health.

ISBN 1-55784-053-8   **$8.95**

3201 S.W. 15th Street,
Deerfield Beach, FL 33442-8190
1-800-851-9100

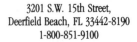 **Health
Communications, Inc.**

Daily Affirmation Books from . . .
Health Communications

TIME FOR JOY: Daily Affirmations
Ruth Fishel

With quotations, thoughts and healing energizing affirmations these daily messages address the fears and imperfections of being human, guiding us through self-acceptance to a tangible peace and the place within where there is *time for joy.*

ISBN 0-932194-82-6 $6.95

SOOTHING MOMENTS: Daily Meditations For Fast-Track Living
Bryan E. Robinson, Ph.D.

This is designed for those leading fast-paced and high-pressured lives who need time out each day to bring self-renewal, joy and serenity into their lives.

ISBN 1-55874-075-9 $6.95

SURVIVING DIVORCE: Daily Affirmations
Sefra Kobrin Pitzele

Surviving Divorce: Daily Affirmations offers sensible advice and affirmations to help ease the pain and restore confidence and self-esteem to those who have suffered a relationship break up.

ISBN 1-55874-118-6 $6.95

GENTLE REMINDERS FOR CO-DEPENDENTS: Daily Affirmations
Mitzi Chandler

With insight and humor, Mitzi Chandler takes the co-dependent and the adult child through the year. *Gentle Reminders* is for those in recovery who seek to enjoy the miracle each day brings.

ISBN 1-55874-020-1 $6.95

AFFIRMATIONS FOR THE INNER CHILD
Rokelle Lerner

This book contains powerful messages and helpful suggestions aimed at adults who have unfinished childhood issues. By reading it daily we can end the cycle of suffering and move from pain into recovery.

ISBN 1-55874-045-6 $6.95

3201 S.W. 15th Street,
Deerfield Beach, FL 33442-8190
1-800-441-5569

Health
Communications, Inc.

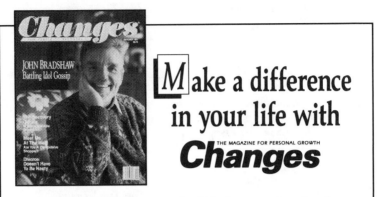